SELECTED TOPICS IN MIDWIFERY CARE

Edited by **Ana Polona Mivšek**

Selected Topics in Midwifery Care

http://dx.doi.org/10.5772/intechopen.74444
Edited by Ana Polona Mivšek

Contributors

Johanna Mathibe-Neke, Suzan Masitenyane, Thembelihle Sylvia Patience Ngxongo, Ruth Turnquist Mielke, Rosemary Ogu, Vetty Agala, Fru Angwafo, Pamela Chirwa Banda, Sama Dohbit, Betty Anane-Fenin, Ufuoma Edewor, Ibimonye Porbeni, Omosivie Maduka, Sevde Aksu, John Kuumuori Ganle, Ebenezer Krampah

First published in London, United Kingdom, 2019 by IntechOpen
IntechOpen is the global imprint of INTECHOPEN LIMITED, registered in England and Wales, registration number: 11086078, The Shard, 25th floor, 32 London Bridge Street
London, SE19SG – United Kingdom
Printed in Croatia

British Library Cataloguing-in-Publication Data
A catalogue record for this book is available from the British Library

Additional hard copies can be obtained from orders@intechopen.com

Selected Topics in Midwifery Care, Edited by Ana Polona Mivšek
p. cm.
Print ISBN 978-1-78985-533-3
Online ISBN 978-1-78985-534-0

For EU product safety concerns:
IN TECH d.o.o., Prolaz Marije Krucifikse Kozulić 3, 51000 Rijeka, Croatia,
info@intechopen.com or visit our website at intechopen.com.

Meet the editor

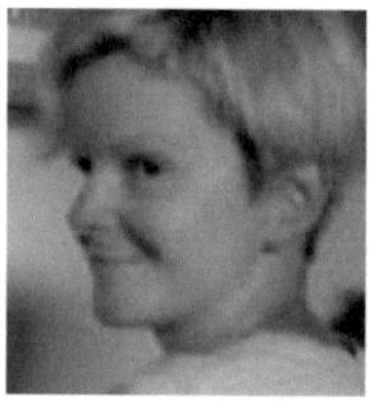

Assistant Professor Ana Polona Mivšek, PhD, is a midwifery teacher at the Faculty of Health Sciences, University of Ljubljana, midwifery department. She finished her BSc in midwifery in Slovenia and her MSc in midwifery in the UK. Her PhD in sociological studies enabled her to have a deeper insight into the current trends of the midwifery profession.
She has worked in the delivery room of the maternity hospital in Ljubljana. Currently, she is lecturing midwifery and sexology in midwifery and teaching practical training to students in connection with physiological and pathological pregnancy.
Besides midwifery she is also interested in combining different knowledge with the aspects of midwifery care, such as psychology, sociology, sexology and ethics. Her primary focus of interest is on preconception health, midwifery care during healthy pregnancy and uncomplicated birth.

Contents

Preface

Midwifery across the globe faces different issues. In some countries the autonomy of the profession is a tradition, while in some societies midwives struggle to practice autonomously the basic competencies. In one part of the world the medicalisation of childbirth is the main issue, preventing the natural processes of pregnancy and childbirth to flow at their own pace, while in other parts of the world midwives struggle with lack of resources to provide safe midwifery care.

The authors of this book practice midwifery in different cultures and within different social contexts. They have to deal with different obstacles and seek solutions to diverse problems. With their contributions, they offer an insight into their thinking, their dilemmas, and the problems of midwifery practices in their countries. However, despite different backgrounds, they all have in common a uniform goal—a wish to offer women optimal midwifery care and to improve midwifery services.

Assist. Prof. Ana Polona Mivšek, PhD
Faculty of Health Sciences
University of Ljubljana, Slovenia

Chapter 1

Basic Antenatal Care Approach to Antenatal Care Service Provision

Thembelihle Sylvia Patience Ngxongo

Additional information is available at the end of the chapter

http://dx.doi.org/10.5772/intechopen.79361

Abstract

Globally, antenatal care is advocated as the cornerstone for reducing children's deaths and improving maternal health. The basic antenatal care approach is used in the public health institutions in South Africa to provide healthcare services to the pregnant women. The basic antenatal care approach is a modified version of the focused antenatal care approach that was recommended by researchers during 2001 and adopted by the World Health Organisation in 2002 following realisation that traditional antenatal care programmes that were meant for developed countries were poorly implemented and largely ineffective when used in developing countries. The basic antenatal care approach is listed as one of the priority interventions for reducing maternal and child mortality in the country and is recommended as the minimum level of antenatal care that every pregnant woman should receive. Every site where pregnant women make contact with healthcare services should provide antenatal care services daily using this approach so that the first antenatal care visit consultation takes place as soon as the pregnancy has been confirmed or the very first time that a pregnant woman visits a health facility. The introductions of the basic antenatal care approach have been a positive milestone for South Africa.

Keywords: antenatal care, approach to health care, basic antenatal care, pregnancy, pregnancy outcome, South Africa

1. Introduction

Antenatal care (ANC) is an umbrella term used to describe medical care and procedures that are carried out to and for the pregnant women [1]. It is the health care that is rendered to the pregnant women throughout pregnancy until the child's birth and is aimed at detecting the already existing problems and/or problems that can develop during pregnancy, affecting the pregnant woman and/or her unborn child [2]. The care includes various screening tests, diagnostic procedures, prophylactic treatments, some of which are done routinely, and others are provided to the women based on identified problems and risk factors.

2. Importance of antenatal care

According to Pattinson [2], ANC benefits both the mother and the baby; it assists in screening, diagnosing and managing or controlling the risk factors that might adversely affect the pregnant women and/or the pregnancy outcome. Maternal and perinatal death rates remain the major challenge of health care in South Africa. During 2005–2007, triennium maternal deaths had increased by 20% when comparing them to the 2002–2004 triennium [3]. However, due to changes in the treatment programmes for HIV-positive pregnant women and the focus on reducing deaths in specific categories such as obstetric haemorrhage, a significant fall in both the numbers of maternal deaths and mortality ratios has since been reported in South Africa. An overall reduction of 24% (1152 from 2008–2010 to 2014–2016) has been achieved [4]. Nevertheless, much more still needs to be done for the country to be able to maintain this fall and to obtain an exponential fall. Several major challenges still remain mainly relating to the quality of care, inter-facility transport, and knowledge and skills of health professionals [4]. Furthermore, the majority of preventable deaths during pregnancy and childbirth have been attributed to poor ANC [5]. According to these authors, non-attendance of ANC clinics carries an approximately four times increased risk of maternal deaths compared with the general pregnant population who attend ANC clinics. The provision of adequate ANC is advocated by most authors worldwide as the cornerstone for maternal and perinatal care. The detection of high-risk pregnancies through ANC has been advocated as a good tool for reducing maternal and perinatal mortality rates [6].

The purpose of ANC is to screen, diagnose and manage or control the risk factors that might adversely affect the pregnant woman and/or the pregnancy outcome. Both Pattinson and Snyman [2, 7] attest to this by saying: 'The quality of health care that a pregnant woman receives during ANC has an impact on the health of the woman and on the outcome of pregnancy'. Ekabua et al. [1] highlight the four major goals of ANC as being (a) promotion and maintenance of the physical and social health of the mother and the baby, (b) detection and management of complications during pregnancy, (c) development of birth preparedness and complication readiness plan and (d) preparation of the women for normal puerperium. The World Health Organisation (WHO) identifies ANC as one of the most widely used strategies to improve maternal and child health [8]. It was also one of the worldwide strategies towards the achievement of millennium development goal (MDGs numbers 4 and 5, which were to reduce child deaths by 75% and improve maternal health by 50% by 2015 [9].

Three South African reports, namely the Saving Mothers report by the National Committee on Confidential Enquiry into Causes of Maternal Deaths (NCCEMD), Saving Babies report for the Perinatal Problem Identification Programme (PPIP) and Saving Children report for the Child Health Problem Identification Programme (CHPIP), review the health care provided to the mothers, babies and children in South Africa [10]. The findings of these reports highlight avoidable causes of the deaths of mothers, babies and children and make recommendations to improve the quality of care provided to mothers, babies and children at the time when they need it most. All three committees highlight, in their triennial reports, the importance of ANC for reducing maternal, perinatal and children's deaths. Bradshaw et al. [10] further emphasise that addressing the health challenges should involve strengthening the provision of healthcare packages within the continuum of care and recognise that the effectiveness of each package depends on whether it provides high-impact, evidence-based interventions and also on the coverage and quality of the service rendered. ANC can screen for, detect and thus prevent many maternal complications that might occur before childbirth and could significantly improve the outcomes for unborn infants [2].

The one document by the NCCEMD, which might appear old but which conveys a very important message for South Africa, is the Saving Mothers Policy and Management Guidelines for Common Causes of Maternal Deaths [11]. This policy document highlights that one of the major areas of substandard care identified in South Africa is the poor initial assessment of patients during ANC visits. The authors attribute this to the fact that the midwives are trained in the traditional method of history taking, clinical examination and special investigations when assessing patients. This might make it difficult to assimilate the multiple abnormalities found and to formulate a management plan for a patient with multiple organ disease, the very type of cases described in the maternity mortality reports [12].

South Africa has a burden of high maternal and perinatal mortality rates and therefore needs to work very hard to address this problem. The number of reported maternal mortalities had increased by 20% during the 2005–2007 triennium compared to the 2002–2004 trienniums [3]. The constant rise in maternal and perinatal mortality rates resulted in South Africa's inclusion of the MNCWH programme as one of the priority programmes in the 10-year strategic plan for the country [12]. The majority of the provider-related preventable deaths in South Africa have been attributed to poor ANC.

South Africa can address the problem of the constantly rising maternal and perinatal mortality rates because the majority of avoidable provider-related maternal deaths can be avoided through providing proper and good-quality ANC services [13]. The Saving Mothers Report 2008–2010 indicates that a total of (16.6%, n = 713) of women who died during this triennium did not attend ANC clinics and (7.0%, n = 300) attended ANC clinics infrequently [14]. The Saving Mothers' Report indicates that the avoidable causes of maternal deaths included a number of health provider-related issues such as poor initial assessments, problems with recognising problems, delays in referring the pregnant women to different healthcare facilities causing pregnant women to be managed at inappropriate healthcare levels, incorrect management, substandard management/care and failure to take actions when abnormalities were found [14].

3. Approaches to antenatal care

Several approaches to ANC are used in different countries including the traditional approach, goal-directed ANC, focussed ANC (FANC) and the basic ANC (BANC) approach. While some countries structure and develop their own approaches to suit their unique circumstances, other countries might simply adopt an approach existing elsewhere. This could create problems if the situations in the two countries differ. Developing countries (like South Africa, Botswana, Swaziland, Kenya and Zimbabwe) adopted ANC programmes modelled on the approaches used in developed countries [15]. These approaches use risk assessments to identify women who are likely to experience complications during their pregnancies and assume that more clinic visits imply better pregnancy outcomes. In these approaches, scarce resources of developing countries might be devoted to women with high-risk pregnancies, implying that women with low-risk pregnancies might not receive optimal care [16]. This approach has been challenged by the WHO [17]. The Maternal and Neonatal Programme [18] argues that frequent ANC visits are often logically and financially impossible for women to manage and place additional burdens on the healthcare system. Frequent ANC visits do not necessarily improve pregnancy outcomes [1]. The WHO realised that traditional ANC programmes, meant for developed countries, were poorly implemented and largely ineffective when used in developing countries [16].

The WHO designed and tested an FANC package that included only counselling, examinations and tests serving an immediate purpose and having a proven health benefit as an ideal approach to be used by developing countries [19]. In the FANC approach, the WHO recommends reducing the number of ANC visits to four, and this has not been found to pose risks to the health of mothers or babies [19]. The FANC approach recognises that every pregnant woman is at risk of experiencing complications and therefore emphasises that all pregnant women should receive the same basic care and monitoring for complications [18]. However, the WHO emphasises that once a pregnant woman has been identified to have high-risk factors, she should be referred to a higher level of care [18]. The WHO therefore advocates that after the initial assessment, pregnant women should be categorised into two groups: those who have low-risk factors who should follow the FANC reduced number of ANC visits approach and those who have high-risk factors who should be referred for hospital management of their pregnancies [19]. The Maternal, Child and Women's Health Unit of the KwaZulu-Natal (KZN) Department of Health reviewed and revised its ANC guidelines on the basis of the WHO's model of FANC to improve the quality of ANC provided at the clinics in the KZN province [20].

According to the MNH Programme [18], the FANC approach is one of several essential maternal and neonatal care interventions that are evidence-based and that build on global lessons learned about saving the lives of mothers and newborn babies. The FANC approach also includes a classifying form designed to assist ANC health-care providers to identify women who have conditions requiring treatment and more frequent monitoring. It also includes classifying forms needed to implement the package and instructions for its use [19].

The WHO provided key recommendations which form standards for maternal and neonatal care service delivery, providing guidance for assisting countries to improve the health and survival of women and newborn babies during pregnancy, childbirth and the postnatal period and can be modified to suit the circumstances of a specific country [21]. These WHO provisions allow each country, intending to adopt the FANC approach, to modify the guidelines to suit the circumstances of the specific country. The WHO indicates that it might be necessary, when introducing the FANC package in practice (depending on the specific country), that the country's national clinical standards and guidelines for ANC might require updating, the pre-service training curricula in ANC and in-service training for ANC providers and their supervisors might need to be modified, and a plan for implementing changes with regard to medications, equipment and supplies to implement the package should be assessed [21].

4. Approaches to antenatal care services in South Africa

Until 2007, South Africa used the traditional approach to ANC. Historically, this traditional ANC service model was developed in the early 1900s. This model assumed that frequent ANC visit, and classifying pregnant women into low- and high-risk groups by predicting potential obstetric complications, was the best way to care for the mother and the foetus [22]. The use of the traditional ANC approach in South Africa was prescribed by the South African Nursing Council (SANC) in the scope of practice for midwives [23]. The SANC prescribed that the midwives should ensure that pregnant women attend ANC clinics once a month until 28 weeks' gestation and thereafter every fortnight until 36 weeks' gestation. Thereafter, a pregnant woman should continue attending the clinic at PHC level every week until her baby is born or until she reached 42 weeks' gestation whichever comes first. Should the woman not give birth by 42 weeks' gestation, she had to be referred for hospital management [23]. With the traditional approach, a pregnant woman could have up to 12 ANC visits conducted at a PHC clinic level during one pregnancy. This is one of the aspects that have been challenged by the WHO [24].

The traditional ANC approach was replaced by the FANC approach which is a goal-oriented ANC approach that was recommended by researchers during 2001 and adopted by the WHO in 2002 [21]. The NDoH identified BANC as the ideal approach to ensure that quality and effective ANC is provided [25]. According to the Saving Babies Report 2008–2009, improvement in access to good-quality ANC services could make a major contribution towards reducing perinatal and child deaths [26].

South Africa adopted and modified the FANC model to suit the South African circumstances and referred to it as the BANC approach [27, 28]. This followed the realisation by the NDoH that the traditional ANC approach was not working well for South Africa. Midwives, the key providers of ANC services, requested for a programme based on the principles used in the Integrated Management of Childhood Illnesses (IMCI) programme with flow diagrams and protocols [2]. In 2007, the NDoH advised that all health facilities providing ANC services had to adopt the BANC approach by the end of 2008 [29]. The BANC approach is used in the public health institutions of South Africa to provide healthcare services to pregnant women and is listed as one of the priority interventions for reducing maternal and child mortality in this country [25]. South Africa's NDoH introduced the BANC approach in 2007 and advised that all health facilities providing antenatal care (ANC) services should have adopted this approach by the end of 2008 [29]. The NDoH provided training for the lead trainers from all the provinces and made available various documents such as a handbook, guidelines and guides for facility managers [2, 28, 29]. The lead trainers were expected to cascade the training into their respective provinces and to institute and facilitate the implementation of the BANC approach.

5. The basic antenatal care (BANC) approach

Pattinson [28] describes the BANC approach as the minimum level of ANC that every pregnant woman should receive. Every aspect of the BANC approach has been developed from the best research evidence, and the only aspects of ANC that have been shown to be effective are included in the BANC approach [28]. The BANC approach does not intend to replace any existing programme but aims to combine all resources and to facilitate their use [28]. The BANC approach was introduced as a quality improvement strategy based on the belief that good-quality ANC could reduce maternal and perinatal mortalities and improve maternal health, aiming to achieve MDGs 4 and 5 [30]. This then led to the introduction of the BANC approach in the PHC clinics. Thus, the BANC was an approach being used in South Africa to render ANC services during the time of this study.

The BANC approach has been simplified to the bare minimum so that ANC services can be provided by every PHC clinic's midwives [28]. Because the BANC approach is a modified version of the FANC approach, it has many characteristics similar to the FANC approach. These include the approach focusing on early ANC attendance by all pregnant women and on limiting the total number of ANC visits to a minimum of four or five visits per pregnancy for low-risk women. This requires that ANC services should be provided daily at every facility frequented by pregnant women so that the first ANC visit takes place as soon as the pregnancy has been confirmed or the very first time that a pregnant woman visits a health facility [28]. If a pregnant woman is brought into the health system early, her health problems could be detected and managed or controlled early and treatment then has a greater chance of success. Pattinson [28] also states that all pregnant women with high-risk factors should be referred to the next level of care so that nurses at PHC level have sufficient time to attend to women with low-risk factors. Every site where pregnant women make contact with health services should be utilised because if all PHC clinics are providing BANC, then ANC could be started as soon as the pregnancy had been confirmed [2].

The BANC approach requires that two sets of checklists be used for recording purposes during ANC visits: one checklist to record the first visit and the other to use during subsequent follow-up visits. Pattinson [28] recommends that before commencing implementation of the BANC approach, each facility has to develop its own specific protocols for the management of obstetric conditions which must be in line with the South African National Maternity Care Guidelines and should be displayed in the facility. All the protocols should be counter-signed by the head of the obstetric unit from the hospital to which the facility refers the women with high-risk factors or complications during pregnancy. The protocols should be reviewed annually. Regular auditing of the ANC service should be an on-going process to ensure continuous improvement based on identifying and addressing potential shortcomings [2].

The BANC approach focuses on the quality rather than on the quantity of visits, with special emphasis on the fact that every visit should be goal directed [31]. The approach is included in the list of strategies provided by the NDoH to achieve MDGs 4 and 5 which are to reduce perinatal deaths and improve maternal health by 2015 [32]. A baseline audit of the ANC service and an analysis of the strengths, weaknesses, opportunities and threats (SWOT) of the facility should be conducted before commencing the implementation of the BANC approach. This enables the midwives to compile a realistic plan and process map for the implementation of the BANC approach [2]. Documents such as the handbook, guidelines and facility manager's guides are available to be used by the midwives during the implementation of the BANC approach [2]. According to the BANC handbook, each clinic should have one or more supervisors to perform the clinical supervision and the administrative tasks [2]. The manager is responsible for providing supportive supervision to the staff members in order to ensure that the clinic's programmes are implemented successfully [2].

6. Provision of antenatal care services according to the basic antenatal care approach

While the BANC approach is adapted from the WHO's FANC model, it is also designed similar to the IMCI programme [2]. This decision was taken in response to the midwives' request for an ANC programme that has flow diagrams and protocols similar to the IMCI programme. The midwives hoped that having such a programme would assist them to render safer and better quality health care to the pregnant women [2]. It is for this reason that the BANC approach is sometimes referred to as the integrated management of pregnancy and childbirth [2, 33].

The NDoH also identified BANC as an ideal approach to ensure that quality and effective ANC is provided [25]. The implementation of BANC is seen as a positive measure to improve the quality of ANC in PHC clinics [7]. Effective and quality ANC could assist South Africa to address the problem of constantly increasing maternal and perinatal mortalities. Snyman [6] stated that the BANC quality improvement package is designed to assist ANC-related clinical management and decision-making at PHC level. This author conducted a qualitative study to assess the effectiveness of the BANC package for improving the quality of ANC services rendered at PHC facilities. With the implementation of the BANC approach, the organisational changes required at the facility level for the improvement of ANC services are facilitated with tools like the integrated flow charts for pregnant women's management, referral protocols and checklists. This could potentially have a positive impact on the outcomes of pregnancies [7].

Guidelines on how to conduct ANC visits are detailed in the Basic Antenatal Care Principles of Good Care and Guidelines [28]. These guidelines have been adapted from a guide for essential practice by the WHO titled 'Pregnancy, Childbirth, Postpartum and Newborn Care' [28]. According to the BANC Principles of Good Care and Guidelines, the principles of good care include communication, workplace and administrative procedures, universal precautions, and cleanliness and organisation of ANC visits [28].

It is stated in the guidelines that communication, privacy and confidentiality during examination and counselling should be ensured at each ANC visit [28]. The importance of service hours, the availability of equipment and drugs, record keeping, and infection prevention and control are highlighted as part of the workplace and administrative procedures [28]. The guidelines describe how the ANC visits should be organised, highlighting that ANC should always begin with rapid assessment and management. All pregnant women, except those with high-risk factors, should have four to five routine ANC visits.

A pregnancy status and birth plan chart, which should be used to assess the pregnant women at each of the four ANC visits, are provided [28]. The chart is used during the first ANC visit to prepare the birth and emergency plan and reviewed and modified according to the need at each subsequent ANC visit. 'Ask, check, look listen and feel' criteria should always be followed during assessments of pregnant women. All pregnant women should be screened for preeclampsia, anaemia, foetal growth and post-maturity at all ANC visits [28]. All women should also be screened for syphilis, Human Immunodeficiency Virus (HIV) and Rhesus factor (RH) [28]. All routine investigations, including the rapid plasma reagent (RPR) test, haemoglobin (Hb) level test, HIV and RH tests should be done using rapid test kits. The guidelines highlight the importance of responding to observed signs and/or problems reported by the pregnant women and contain a guide on how to respond to these signs [28].

Standard preventative therapy, including tetanus toxoid injections, iron preparations and calcium supplements, should be issued to all pregnant women at each ANC [28]. A guide is included on how to advise women about nutrition and self-care [28]. The guidelines highlight the importance of preparing individualised ANC and delivery plans for each woman at the first ANC visit and that the plans should be reviewed during each subsequent visit and adjusted based on the identified needs. The plan should be prepared in consultation with the woman concerned. This ensures that the woman is involved in her own care. The plans should also include transport arrangements, infant feeding options and future contraception. A description of how the first and the follow-up visits should be conducted is provided [28].

The guidelines state that the first ANC visit should take place as early in pregnancy as possible, before 12 weeks' gestation, preferably at the confirmation of pregnancy [28]. During the first ANC visit, all women should be classified for BANC using the classifying form/first visit checklist provided. Only women with low-risk factors should follow the BANC approach. All women with risk factors should either be referred to an appropriate level of care or follow a specially prepared schedule based on the risk factors identified. Four follow-up visits should be scheduled at 20, 26, 32 and 38 weeks' gestation. Specific times are scheduled for performing repeat routine tests such as Hb, HIV and RPR, and these times coincide with specific routine follow-up visits. It is therefore important to schedule the follow-up visits as specified by the BANC guidelines in order to ensure the correct timing of repeat tests.

Pattinson [2] suggests that each PHC clinic should have one or more people in the role of ANC supervisor to ensure clinical and administrative supervision. The clinical supervisor should be the person with most ANC skills and should check each pregnant woman's ANC card at the first visit and again at the 32 weeks' visit to ensure that the clinic provides adequate care [2].

All information regarding pregnancy and consultation should be recorded in an ANC card which should not be filed at the clinic but which should be kept by the pregnant woman. The woman is advised to always carry the ANC card with her, wherever she goes, and to produce the card each time she visits any health-care institution. This practice facilitates communication between the different health-care providers involved in the care of women during pregnancy and childbirth [2].

7. Discussion

Several factors have been identified to be positively influencing the implementation of the BANC approach. These include the availability and accessibility of BANC services, policies, guidelines and protocol; various means of communication; a comprehensive package of and the integration of primary healthcare services; training and in-service education; human and material resources; the support and supervision offered to the midwives by the primary health-care supervisors; supervisors' understanding of the approach and the levels of experience of midwives involved in the implementation of the BANC approach [34] Nevertheless, evidence still shows that not all PHC clinics have been able to successfully implement and sustain the BANC approach [35]. Ngxongo [35] discovered that out of 59 Municipal PHC clinics in eThekwini District in KwaZulu-Natal, 46% (n = 27) were successfully implementing the BANC approach. Midwives face various challenges during the implementation of the BANC approach which has resulted in some PHC clinics abandoning the BANC approach and reverting to the traditional approach to ANC [35]. These challenges include shortage of staff, lack of cooperation from referral hospitals, lack of in-service training, problems with transportation of specimens to laboratories, lack of material resources, unavailability of Basic Antenatal Care programme guidelines and lack of management support [35].

Although the BANC approach emphasises quality over quantity of visits [36], reducing the number of ANC visits has posed numerous challenges in the pregnancy outcomes. According to Hofmeyr and Mentrop [37], too few visits and the long interval between routine ANC visits in late pregnancy in the BANC approach have been responsible for a number of maternal and perinatal deaths. Hofmeyr and Mentrop [37] argue that the more frequent and closely spaced ANC visits as pregnancy advances in the traditional approach assisted in early diagnosis and management of selected ANC problems such as preeclampsia, foetal growth impairment and others and that too few visits result in missed opportunities to detect and treat asymptomatic pregnancy complications. These authors recommend modification of the BANC approach into what they call 'BANC plus'. Their proposal is that a reasonable compromise for a middle-income country such as South Africa would be to continue to implement the WHO BANC approach with reduced, goal-orientated visits up to 32 weeks' gestation and thereafter to revert to routine visits every 2–36 or 38 weeks, followed by weekly checks.

The international evidence supports a more regular contact between healthcare workers and pregnant women. Therefore, South Africa is gradually switching to an eight-contact model (three more visits than the current five contact Basic Antenatal Care (BANC) policy) [38]. It is envisaged that this intervention will improve the pregnancy experience as well as the outcomes of pregnant women and their babies in South Africa. The BANC + continues to emphasise the importance of conducting the first visit as early as possible, with the next visit scheduled at 20 weeks and then repeat visits at 26 weeks. The adjustments include the 30 weeks and 34 weeks and then a 2-week visit until delivery. An audit of the current BANC system has shown that two important principles of good care were often missing: a plan for further antenatal care and the delivery plan (including delivery at the appropriate level of care or hospital). Therefore, appropriate planning for the pregnancy as well as for the delivery, based on information obtained and correctly interpreted at every visit, will ensure that women and their families are ready and prepared when the big day arrives. The purpose of BANC+ is not just to increase the number of visits but also an opportunity to look again at how that care is given [38].

8. Conclusion

The introduction of the BANC approach has been a positive milestone for South Africa. Studies show that many African countries such as Ghana, Kenya, Tanzania and others have seen positive results with the implementation of the WHO FANC model [1, 8, 17]. Although South Africa is still experiencing numerous challenges with the BANC approach, there is hope that this country will also achieve positive results as the country continues to adjust and improve the BANC approach to suit its circumstances.

Acknowledgements

The author would like to acknowledge the following: Prof. NS Sibiya and Prof. NS Gwele; Durban University of Technology; SANTRUST, Fundisa and NRF.

Conflict of interest

The author declares that she has no financial or personal relationship which may have inappropriately influenced her in writing this chapter.

Author details

Thembelihle Sylvia Patience Ngxongo

Address all correspondence to: thembelihlen@dut.ac.za

Durban University of Technology, KwaZulu-Natal, South Africa

References

[1] Ekabua J, Ekabua K, Njoku C. Proposed framework for making focussed antenatal care services accessible: A review of the Nigerian setting. ISRN Obstetrics and Gynecology. 2011. DOI: 10.5402/2011/253964

[2] Pattinson RC. Basic Antenatal Care Handbook. Pretoria: University of Pretoria; 2007

[3] National Committee on Confidential Enquiry into Causes of Maternal Deaths. Saving Mothers 2005-2007: Fourth Report on Confidential Enquiries into Maternal Deaths in South Africa. Pretoria: National Department of Health; 2009

[4] National Committee on Confidential Enquiry into Causes of Maternal Deaths. Saving Mothers 2014-2016: Seventh Report on Confidential Enquiries into Maternal Deaths in South Africa. Pretoria: National Department of Health; 2017

[5] National Committee on Confidential Enquiry into Causes of Maternal Deaths. Saving Mothers 2002-2004: Third Report on Confidential Enquiries into Maternal Deaths in South Africa. Pretoria: National Department of Health; 2005

[6] Hoque MM, Hoque E, Kader S. Audit of antenatal care in a rural district of KZN, South Africa. South African Family Practice. 2008;**50**:66

[7] Snyman JS. Effectiveness of the basic antenatal care package in primary health care clinics [Magister Curationis dissertation thesis]. Port Elizabeth: Nelson Mandela Metropolitan University; 2007

[8] World Health Organization. Antenatal Care in Developing Countries: Promises Achievements and Missed Opportunities. An analysis of trends level and differentials 1999-2001 [Internet]. 2003. Available from: http://www.childinfo.org/files/antenatal_care.pd [Accessed: 2014-07-04]

[9] National Department of Health (of South Africa). MRC unit for maternal and infant care strategies, PPIP users, and saving babies technical task team. 2007: Saving Babies 2003-2005 Fifth Report on Perinatal Care in South Africa. Pretoria: Government Printer; 2007

[10] Bradshaw D, Copra M, Kerber K, Lawn J, Moodley J, Pattinson J, Patrick M, Stephen C, Velaphi S. Every Death Counts: Saving the Lives of Mothers, Babies and Children in South Africa. Cape Town: Mills Litho; 2008

[11] National Committee on Confidential Enquiry into Causes of Maternal Deaths. Saving Mothers Policy and Management Guidelines for Common Causes of Maternal Deaths. Pretoria; 2001

[12] South Africa: National Department of Health. National Department of Health. National Department of Health strategic plan 2010; 2010//11-2012/13

[13] Chandni JCS, Hodgson R, Hayen A. Factors associated with the use and quality of antenatal care in Nepal: A population-based study using the demographic and health survey data. BioMed Central Pregnancy and Childbirth. 2014;**14**:94

[14] National Committee on Confidential Enquiry into Causes of Maternal Deaths. Saving Mothers 2008-2010: Fifth Report on Confidential Enquiries into Maternal Deaths in South Africa. Pretoria: National Department of Health; 2012

[15] Villar J, Carroli G, Khan-Neelofur D, Piaggo G, Gulmezoglu M. Patterns of routine antenatal care for low-risk pregnancies: Database of systematic review [Internet]. 2007. Available from: www.who.int/rhl/reviews/langs/CD000934.pdf [Accessed: 2013-08-09]

[16] The Free Library Population brief: Focussed ANC acceptable, tricky to implement [Internet]. 2007. Available from: www.popcouncil.org/uploads/pdfs/.../RH_Focussed AntenatalCare_A4.pdf [Accessed: 2013-02-02]

[17] Mathole T, Lindmark G, Ahlberg BM. Dilemmas and paradoxes in providing and changing antenatal care. Health Policy and Planning. 2005;**20**(6):385-393. DOI: 10.1093/heapol/czi046

[18] Maternal and Neonatal Health Programme. Focused antenatal care: Planning and providing care during pregnancy. [Internet]. 2004. Available from: www.mnh.jhpiego.org [Accessed: 2004-09-21]

[19] World Health Organization. WHO Programme to Map Best Reproductive Health Practices—WHO Antenatal Care Randomized Trial: Manual for Implementation of the New Model. Geneva: WHO; 2002

[20] Population Council. Adapting focussed antenatal lessons from three African countries. Program Brief No. 11. July 2008. [Internet]. 2008. Available from: www.popcouncil.org/uploads/pdfs/frontiers/pbriefs/PB11.pdf [Accessed: 2013-08-28]

[21] World Health Organization. Standards for maternal and neonatal care: Making pregnancy safer [Internet]. 2007. Available from: www.who.int/reproductivehealth/publications/maternal...health/.../en/ [Accessed: 2014-07-09]

[22] Ethiopia Health Education and Training (HEAT) Module. Antenatal Care Ethiopia HEAT Module [Internet]. 2004. Available from: www.open.edu/openlearnworks/mod/oucontent/view.php?id=28 [Accessed: 2014-10-19]

[23] South African Nursing Council. R2598. Regulations relating to the scope of practice of persons who are registered or enrolled [Internet]. 1991. Available from: www.sanc.co.za/regulat/Reg-scp.htm [Accessed: 2013-07-08]

[24] Pell C, Menaca A, Were F, Afrah NA, Chatio S, Manda-Taylo L, Hamel MJ, Hogson A, Tagbor H, Kalilani L, Ouma P, Pool R. Factors affecting antenatal care attendance: Results from qualitative studies in Ghana, Kenya and Malawi. PLoS One. 2013;**8**(1):e53747. DOI: 10.1371/journal.pone.0053747

[25] National Department of Health (of South Africa). Strategic plan for maternal, newborn, child and women's health (MNCWH) and nutrition in South Africa 2012-2016 [Internet]. 2012. Available from: www.doh.gov.za/docs/stratdocs/2012/MNCWHstratplan.pdf [Accessed: 2014-10-13]

[26] National Department of Health (of South Africa). MRC Unit for Maternal and Infant Care Strategies, PPIP Users, and Saving Babies Technical Task Team. Saving Babies 2008-2009 Sixth Report on Perinatal Care in South Africa. Pretoria: Government Printer; 2010

[27] Beksinska M, Kunene B, Mullick S. Maternal care: Antenatal, peri and postnatal: Women's health. In: Ijumba P, Padarath A, editors. South African Health Review. Durban: Health Systems Trust. ISSN 102517515 [Internet]. Available from: http://www.hst.org.za/uploads/files/chap18_06.pdf; 2006. pp. 297-314 [Accessed: 2013-06-18]

[28] Pattinson RC. Basic Antenatal Care Principles of Good Care and Guidelines. Pretoria: University of Pretoria; 2005

[29] Pattinson RC. Basic Ante Natal Care: Facility manager's Notes. Pretoria: University of Pretoria; 2005

[30] National Department of Health (of South Africa). Framework for Accelerating Community-Based Maternal, Neonatal, Child and women's Health and Nutrition Interventions. Pretoria: Government Printer; 2008

[31] National Department of Health (of South Africa). Maternity Case Record Guidelines. Pretoria: Government Printer; 2008

[32] National Department of Health (of South Africa). Guidelines for Maternity Care in South Africa. A Manual for Clinics, Community Health Care Centres and District Hospitals. 3rd ed. Pretoria: Government Printer; 2007

[33] Mhlanga E. Maternal, Newborn and Child Health: 30 Years on. [Internet]. 2012. Available from: www.hst.org.za/uploads/files/chap8 08.pdf [Accessed: 2013-07-08]

[34] Ngxongo TSP. Factors influencing successful implementation of basic antenatal care in eThekwini district [thesis M. Tech dissertation]. Durban: Durban University of Technology; 2011

[35] Ngxongo TSP, Sibiya MN. Challenges regarding the implementation of basic antenatal care in eThekwini district, KwaZulu-Natal. Journal of Nursing. 2013;**22**(7):906-913

[36] Kinze B, Gomez P. Basic Maternal and Newborn Car: A Guide for Skilled Providers. Baltimore, MD: JHPIEGO/MNH Program; 2004

[37] Hofmeyr GJ, Mentrop L. Time for 'basic antenatal care plus' in South Africa? South African Medical Journal. 2015;**105**(11):902-903. DOI: 10.7196/SAMJ.2015.v105i11.10186

[38] World Health Organization. What's new? Decreasing deaths during pregnancy in South Africa by improving antenatal care [Internet]. 2018. Available from: www.who.int [Accessed: 2018-02-11]

Chapter 2

Psychosocial Antenatal Care: A Midwifery Context

Johanna Mmabojalwa Mathibe-Neke and
Seipati Suzan Masitenyane

Additional information is available at the end of the chapter

http://dx.doi.org/10.5772/intechopen.80394

Abstract

The rationale of any national screening programme is to recognise the benefits for public health, to assess a predominantly healthy population including pregnant women and to detect risk factors for morbidity in order to provide timely care interventions. The focus of antenatal care screening is to identify wider determinants of health that may have an impact on a pregnant woman's well-being that includes the physical, psychological, social and religious factors. Psychosocial risks, among others, include poor socioeconomic conditions such as poverty, lack of social support, general health inequalities, domestic violence and a history of either personal or familial mental illness, all of which have the capacity to influence a pregnant woman's decision to utilise health care services. This chapter highlights the antenatal care process, the importance of psychosocial care during pregnancy, maternal risks during pregnancy, the impact of pregnancy on maternal well-being, the possible psychosocial risk factors during pregnancy, psychosocial assessment, psychosocial care as a missing piece of the antenatal care puzzle, the presentation of the results of a study on psychosocial risk assessment and support and further outlining various antenatal care approaches that could be adopted to offer pregnant women holistic care.

Keywords: antenatal care screening, pregnancy, psychosocial care, psychosocial support, women

1. Introduction

This chapter presents a discussion pertaining to psychosocial care for women during pregnancy. Pregnancy as a developmental phase involves both physiological and psychological adaptations that are acceptable to a certain extent, but if excessive, may lead to pathological changes. Psychosocial stressors experienced during pregnancy encompass life experiences that include changes in personal life, job status, family makeup, housing and the possibility of domestic violence [1]. While risks cannot be totally eliminated once pregnancy is established, they can be reduced through effective, accessible and affordable maternity health care. Numerous studies reveal significant depressive symptoms in pregnant women that are associated with sociodemographic and economic status and that depression during pregnancy may negatively influence psychosocial adjustment [2, 3]. Research findings also recommend an integrated approach to antenatal care that focuses on both the physiological and psychosocial dimensions.

2. Antenatal care as a process

Antenatal care has been described as one of the effective forms of preventative care. It involves screening symptomatic and asymptomatic pregnant women, with the aim of detecting and thereby preventing both maternal and neonatal adverse events. The introduction of antenatal care in 1910 in the Royal Adelaide Hospital in Australia has played an important role in preventing high maternal and perinatal mortality rates. Antenatal care should ideally be geared towards the promotion of health and the prevention of physical and psychosocial problems [16].

The psychopathology of pregnancy needs to be understood in terms of the adjustment that all women have to make when they conceive, as pregnancy is also an adaptive process. A pregnant woman should carry the baby safely through to delivery and adjust to the sacrifices that motherhood demands. The challenges that face her, include the acceptance of the pregnancy by the family; development of an attachment to the baby and preparation for birth; and adjustment to the changes in her physical appearance, and to development and maintenance of a positive relationship with the father of the baby. Many women respond to this complex process with grief and anger, especially when the pregnancy is unplanned and unaccepted. Unmanaged grief or anger might ultimately lead to maternal depression [17].

Pregnancy can be enhanced through a coordinated antenatal care programme, which includes both medical and psychosocial care. As such, pregnant women's mental health should be a primary concern for all midwives due to a reported high prevalence of depressive and anxiety disorders in women. Hollander and Langer [18, 19] reported a 21% incidence of depression and 34% anxiety disorders in women, which may be exacerbated by pregnancy. Pregnancy-specific anxiety may occur as the woman worries about her pregnancy, physical changes and delivery.

Antenatal preparation should be offered to all women during pregnancy as a national policy. Screening during pregnancy is crucial, with the aim of detecting and preventing both maternal and neonatal adverse events and instituting early intervention. During screening, midwives should actively listen to the concerns and needs of pregnant women to be able to assess them comprehensively.

The findings of a cross-cultural survey by Namagembe [20] on the extent of physical and emotional abuse on African American, White American and Hispanic women during pregnancy indicated that one in four women gave a history of battering and physical abuse. The implication for this was that many women's community subsystems of safety and physical environment are not in harmony and that battering and physical abuse during pregnancy might lead to a significant delay in obtaining antenatal care by 6.5 weeks as compared to non-abused women.

http://dx.doi.org/10.5772/intechopen.80394

During childbirth, women may look upon their midwives as their advocates despite the existing medically inclined maternity care context. The challenge faced by midwives is the provision of comprehensive and holistic maternity care. This challenge can be achieved through the maintenance of a woman-centred, individualised and caring approach, which needs a caring and responsive midwife. Midwifery care should involve the physical, emotional, social, spiritual and psychological elements for it to be regarded as comprehensive [14].

3. The importance of psychosocial care during pregnancy

Psychosocial morbidity is not given enough recognition, it is not thought to be self-limiting as it is the care that is attributed to normal emotionality of pregnancy, and it is less frequently identified, especially if there is no continuity of care by the same midwife or clinician. Pereira et al. [4] reported that antenatal depression affects 4–16% of women, domestic violence during pregnancy rates at 16% and postnatal depression affects 15–20% of postpartum women.

Historically and contemporarily [4], much of what constitutes antenatal care throughout the world remains strongly rooted in the medical model within which it developed. Widespread, institutionalised routine antenatal care began around 80 years ago, focusing on mass screening with the aim of reducing maternal and perinatal morbidity and mortality under medical supervision [5] What is of concern within the context of antenatal care are the beliefs and assumptions that continue to underpin the structure and content of antenatal care.

Traditionally, antenatal care consists of a prescribed set of acts with a focus on the clinical physiological monitoring and screening of pregnant women. This approach was based on the notion by Oakley (1984) that pregnancy is a state of pathology rather than a normal physiological and developmental stage [5]. As further stated by Chitra and Gnanadurai [1], "antenatal care is usually offered in a form of routine physical assessment and care with limited or no psychosocial assessment and care".

Inadequate psychosocial risk assessment may lead to lack of psychosocial support afforded to the pregnant women. Pregnant women who lack psychosocial support may experience stress during their pregnancy and childbirth. These changes may increase the woman's vulnerability to depression, which may in turn have adverse effects on both maternal and foetal well-being [6]. Unrelieved stress can also increase vulnerability to physical and emotional problems, for example, insomnia, fatigue, development of ulcers and heart problems [7].

Supportive care during childbirth may have long-term positive effects and may protect some women from a long-lasting negative birth experience. The latter was found in a longitudinal cohort study on "why some women change their opinions about childbirth over time" [8]. Mixed feelings were elicited from women regarding their attitude towards childbirth, changing from positive to less-positive opinions based on, for instance, dissatisfaction with intrapartum care and lack of support for psychosocial problems such as single marital status or the presence of depressive symptoms. Changing from negative to less-negative feelings was associated with less worry about birth in early pregnancy and a more positive experience of support by the midwife.

According to O'Keane and Marsh [9], psychosocial support not only lowers prematurity and low birth weight rates but also inspires healthier behaviours and lifestyle among pregnant women and discourages behaviours like smoking, substance abuse and poor nutritional intake, which can have other detrimental effects on the mother and baby. Psychosocial support calls for a multi-level approach, consisting of strengthening partners and families and enhancing system capacity by ensuring the availability of resources. Interventions need to bolster the support provided within the woman's existing social network in order to maintain the woman's cultural beliefs and values.

Dodd et al. [10] tested a hypothesis on the relationship between psychosocial stress, social support, self-efficacy and circulating pro- and anti-inflammatory cytokines in women throughout pregnancy. Pregnant women within the study completed the Denver Maternal Health Assessment. The conclusion was that high social support was associated with low stress scores. Elevated stress scores positively correlated with higher levels of pro-inflammatory cytokine interleukin-6 (IL-6) and tumour necrosis factor-α (TNF-α).

A longitudinal community-based study conducted by Gelder et al. [11] through the use of the Edinburgh Postnatal Depression Scale (EPDS) revealed that women who lacked social support showed more symptoms of depressed mood. The maternal depressive mood had a negative impact on breastfeeding, the experiences of motherhood and the relationship with partners.

Appropriate psychosocial assessment is important for designing relevant intervention strategies and for public health policy formulation [12]. Ethically, psychosocial risk assessment should be linked to a plan of care through the provision of appropriate psychosocial support. The plan of care should ensure that the maternal referral arrangements are in place at the participating facilities. The plan of care should be coordinated with all appropriate disciplines.

Irrespective of how maternity care providers perceive antenatal care, the important issue to be taken into consideration is the woman. From a psychosocial point of view, for midwives using a midwifery model, antenatal care is a time of building a relationship with each woman and her family. It is a time when a partnership is developed and negotiated; expectations, roles and responsibilities are identified; options are discussed and choices are made by women and supported by midwives.

While not neglecting physical safety, antenatal care should be emotionally, socially, culturally and religiously acceptable to the woman. Physical care alone is not sufficient for the woman, as her needs and expectations are unique. The effectiveness of antenatal care as a central focus is still being discussed by midwives, obstetricians, medical anthropologists, sociologists and women's organisations. Handley [13] cited Oakley (1984) in her book "Captured Womb" and wrote extensively on pregnancy, antenatal care and childbirth. She argues the importance of antenatal care but also believes that antenatal care is something that is done in an attempt to control the behaviour of women's bodies, an intervention offered to women that does not benefit all women, but probably a few who do not know what to expect from an antenatal care service.

Purdy (2001) as cited by Woodward [14] defines medicalisation as the process that transpires when health practitioners treat natural bodily functions as if they were diseased. Purdy further stated that it is essential that conventional medicine re-evaluates its health care model towards the needs of patients and not its own.

Conventional medicine must also accept other health care practices such as midwifery-led maternity care as a valid source of healthcare, especially to address psychosocial risk factors. Women's health problems, including pregnancy, should cease to be medicalised.

Parry [15] in a study exploring whether Canadian women's choice of midwifery care identifies a resistance to the medicalisation of pregnancy and childbirth came to the conclusion that women have a desire for personal control of their pregnancy as reflected in this comment:

> *"I just wanted to be in control of what was going on with my body, It scares me that they will push you when you are in your most vulnerable state, because it is more convenient for their schedule". Participants further related how midwifery care met their needs for control over their bodies, their pregnancies and their experiences with childbirth, notwithstanding a sentiment that medical interventions also have a place in pregnancy and childbirth.*

An ideal option for effective antenatal care is the incorporation of psychosocial care as a component of antenatal care, acknowledging the women's own experiences of pregnancy [2]. Midwifery, which means "to be with women", is based upon a philosophy of care in which the management of pregnancy is shared between the midwife and the woman, with a focus on informed choice, shared responsibility, mutual decision making and women articulating their health needs.

4. Maternal risks during pregnancy

According to Baldo [7], maternal risk is defined as the probability of experiencing various levels of injuries or even dying as a result of pregnancy or childbirth. Physiological and psychosocial risk screening should therefore be conducted during the first and subsequent visits of antenatal care as part of a comprehensive assessment during antenatal care.

The opinions of Handwerker (1994), Lupton (1999) and Saxell (2000) as cited by Refs. [1, 21] were that risk assessment during childbirth is made more complex by the differences in the perceptions of risks between midwives and pregnant women, as risk from a midwife's perspective is based on her specialised knowledge and training, epidemiology, personal values and experience, whereas a woman's understanding of risk is far more contextual, individualised and embedded in her social environment and everyday life experience.

Historically, the definition of maternal risk emphasises mainly medical factors and includes few psychological and socioeconomic factors. To add to this, the interest of midwives seems to be directed towards foetal well-being and the newborn child, ignoring the psychosocial needs of the mother. Furthermore, when a woman reports for delivery, her family member's concern is mostly on the well-being of the newborn rather than on the maternal well-being.

Psychosocial factors are an important area to assess during pregnancy. Various studies, for example, those of [12, 22–24] demonstrate that stress, depression, alcohol abuse and lack of social support during pregnancy are commonly associated with low birth weight and perinatal morbidity and mortality. Furthermore, in this era of HIV/AIDS, psychosocial problems are common among affected populations. These issues may have an indirect influence by affecting antenatal care attendance, the woman's coping capacity and the physiology of pregnancy.

Most of the risk assessment systems in midwifery care focuses on physical characteristics such as age, parity and education; however, these assessment systems are not exclusively suggestive of a risk for maternal morbidity and mortality as they mostly exclude psychosocial factors. A review of several studies by Hamid et al. [25] on the perceptions of antenatal care by women suggests that there are several psychosocial risk factors that need to be taken into consideration in order to ensure a safe pregnancy and delivery. Psychosocial interventions have proved to be beneficial in providing comprehensive antenatal care.

Furthermore, a systematic review of 16 studies on antenatal screening for postnatal depression by Hamid et al. [25], which involved 23,000 participants, revealed that the proportion of women who are at risk for postnatal depression was between 10 and 67%. The authors further commented that the preliminary evidence suggested that the introduction of screening tools to aid early detection and diagnosis of depression has helped to raise awareness among health care providers regarding social and psychological maternal risk factors.

5. Possible psychosocial risk factors during pregnancy

Psychosocial risks are described as the demands or challenges that are psychological or social in origin, having the potential to directly or indirectly alter homeostasis during pregnancy and childbirth [21]. They relate to a combination of the affective states and cognitive factors of anxiety, depression, self-esteem mastery and perceived stress as measured by the scale of Gunn et al. [30].

According to Glazier et al. [28], a psychosocial problem may occur in response to an exposure to a stressful life event, for example, unemployment. The psychosocial response will, however, be determined by the effect it has on an individual, for example, loss of self-esteem and feelings of worthlessness.

Fawole et al. [29] have identified the following as some of the psychosocial risk factors that a woman may have experienced or may experience during pregnancy: woman battering; family violence or intimate partner abuse; sexual abuse and harassment; discrimination; gender inequality; past history of depressive disorders; absent/abusive or non-supportive spouse; marital difficulties; pregnancy occurring below 18 years of age, which antedates social development; unintended, unplanned or unwanted pregnancy; maternal or paternal unemployment; adverse life events, for example, loss of spouse; socio-economic factors, for example, poverty; barriers to accessing health care services, for example, distance travelled and transport unavailability; medical disorders, for example, hypertension and HIV/AIDS and poor quality of interaction with health care providers that may lead to non-compliance to planned interventions and defaulting treatment.

6. The impact of pregnancy on maternal well-being

6.1. The physiological effect of pregnancy

Pregnancy may have an enormous psychological and physiological effect on a woman's body and mind. This is due to suppression of the hypothalamic-pituitary-adrenal axis, which leads to dramatic changes in oestrogen and progesterone levels. Changes in these hormone levels may alter a pregnant woman's coping mechanisms. The physical discomfort of pregnancy, accompanied by anticipation of childbirth and the responsibility of parenthood, often causes anxiety and emotional changes [27].

6.2. Stress alters physiology

There is a growing body of data suggesting that psychosocial factors such as high stress and low social support negatively affect the success of pregnancy. The findings of a survey by Shamim ul Moula [26] to address relationships between psychosocial variables and serum inflammatory markers during pregnancy support the notion that prenatal stress alters maternal physiology and immune function in a manner that is consistent with an increased risk of pregnancy complications such as preterm delivery and pregnancy-induced hypertension. The conclusion based on the findings of the above survey was a need for the development of strategies for supporting maternal mental health.

6.3. The impact of psychosocial stress on maternal and foetal well-being

It is clear that birth and infant development are affected by prenatal events that could lead to maternal stress. Maternal psychosocial stress has been recently identified as a factor in early foetal development. There is growing evidence that perinatal psychological and environmental stressors are detrimental to pregnancy success and infant outcomes. Stress is often defined as events, situations, emotions and interactions that are perceived as negatively affecting the well-being of an individual or that cause responses that are perceived as harmful [10].

A direct relationship is said to exist between maternal psychological stress and low birth weight, prematurity and intra-uterine growth retention. This is related to the release of catecholamines that results in placental hypo-perfusion and consequent restriction of oxygen and inhibition of nutrients to the foetus, leading to foetal growth impairment [27].

6.4. The relationship between antenatal depression and postnatal depression

There is considerable evidence that postnatal depression is a public health care challenge as it can become chronic, can damage the relationship between the woman and her partner and might have adverse consequences for the emotional and cognitive development of the newborn. Regular assessment of mood during pregnancy should be routine for all women to establish the risk for depression, as postnatal depression can recur. Antenatal mood assessment is one of the most robust predictors of postnatal depression, as 50% of postnatal depression is reported to have begun during pregnancy [27].

There is evidence from research that women with antenatal psychosocial risk factors are more likely to have a postnatal mood disorder, and as such, antenatal assessment can be beneficial for these women. The early identification and management of psychosocial risk factors have been shown to be beneficial in various studies. For example, in the study by Ref. [29], regarding the review of existing tools that are used to assess psychosocial morbidity in pregnant women, and a study by Gunn et al. [30] on anxiety and depression during pregnancy, outcomes were improved by minimising the occurrence of postpartum depression.

Recommendations from a survey by Namagembe [20] were that a search for battering and abuse should be carried out during the antenatal assessment of pregnant women and midwives should have knowledge of the appropriate interventions and be familiar with the resources for referral. The increased cost and complications that may arise as a result of any delays should be a concern for maternal-child health professionals. Routine antenatal and postnatal screening for psychosocial distress has been supported by investigators as a preventive measure for postnatal depression [28].

7. Psychosocial assessment

Psychosocial assessment is defined by Chitra and Gnanadurai [1] as an evaluation of an individual's mental health, social status and functional capacity. The individual's physical status, appearance and modes of behaviour are observed for factors that may indicate or contribute to emotional distress or mental illness. Observation includes posture, facial expressions, manner of dress, speech and thought patterns, degree of motor activity and level of consciousness. The individual is questioned concerning patterns of daily living, including work schedule and social and leisure activities. Data should include the individual's response to and methods of coping with stress, relationships, cultural orientation, unemployment or change of employment, change of residence, marriage, divorce or death of a loved one [30].

The above-listed risk factors can directly or indirectly affect the outcome of pregnancy in a negative way [7]. A meta-analysis of perinatal depression identified depression as a major complication of pregnancy affecting 14.5% of pregnant women [19].

8. Psychosocial care as a missing piece of the antenatal care puzzle

Traditionally and in many contemporary contexts, including in South Africa, antenatal care consists of a prescribed set of acts based around the clinical monitoring and screening of all pregnant women. This establishment of routine care was based on the notion that pregnancy is a state of pathology rather than normal physiology. There is evidence of a focus on technological dominance and a focus on the detection of obstetric and medical conditions occurring during pregnancy. This is based on a review of seven guidelines for antenatal care from the USA, Canada, Australia and Germany and mostly reflects expert opinion rather than scientific evidence [21].

For example, antenatal care in South Africa is provided at the primary, secondary and tertiary levels of care in both the public and private health care systems. Basic antenatal care services include physical examination, weight measurement, urinalysis, blood pressure monitoring, blood investigations and health information and are supposedly provided at all levels of antenatal care as routine practice.

The ongoing debate on antenatal care regarding its frequency, content, continuity, quality and effectiveness in reducing maternal and neonatal morbidity and mortality led to a new evidence-based protocol on the frequency of antenatal care. This is the result of randomised trials carried out in the United Kingdom and Zimbabwe and of the World Health Organisation trials in Thailand, Argentina, Cuba and Saudi Arabia during 1996 [31].

The new schedule, as recommended by WHO [30], consists of four visits during pregnancy, the first one being early in pregnancy, with subsequent visits at 26, 32 and 36 weeks. This schedule is designed for the pregnant woman at low risk. These fewer antenatal visits led to poorer psychosocial outcomes and drew attention to greater maternal satisfaction with the routine care that was previously provided. The question is whether there would be an opportunity for the midwives to address psychosocial care within this regime.

Baldo [7] in a review of the antenatal care debate quoted Mcllwaine (1980) highlighting that he was amazed that pregnant women came for antenatal care and waited in the clinic for 2 hours, only to be seen for 2 minutes by someone laying his or her hands on them, and then leave. The reason for this is the traditional focus on the biophysiology of pregnancy. The author recommended that antenatal care appointments should be structured, focused and advocated for longer first appointments to allow comprehensive assessment in order to address both physiological and psychosocial risk factors.

The Changing Childbirth report explicitly confirmed that women should be the focus of antenatal care to enable a woman to make informed decisions based on her needs, having discussed her matters with the midwife involved. Key aspects of care valued by women are reported to be respect, competence, communication, support and convenience [32].

The above are supported by the researcher's findings from a phenomenological study on the expectations of antenatal care by pregnant women. Most women were happy with the physical health care but were dissatisfied with interpersonal aspects, for example, involvement, guidance and communication from the health care providers [33].

As a midwifery lecturer, the researcher often accompanied students for clinical facilitation. On guiding students on psychosocial care of women in the antenatal care clinic, women frequently verbalised social and emotional concerns. The researcher's further experience is that if psychosocial assessment is indeed conducted on a pregnant woman, it usually elicits the woman's current active and significant psychosocial challenges.

The following are common remarks that were expressed by women during their antenatal visits while the researcher was engaged in student accompaniment.

A woman carrying her first pregnancy at age 25, gravida 1 para 0, from one of Gauteng's provincial hospital's antenatal clinic remarked:

> *"No one ever asked me this. Why don't everyone do like this? I think I am lucky today, I had so much to ask or discuss previously but there was just no one to listen to me. I moved from a black hospital to a one for whites thinking things will be better but it's the same. We come here, they quickly check the baby, and within 30 minutes you are gone with so much to share, as if the baby is the only one important". She then asked for the lecturer's and the student's contact numbers for further consultation.*

A pregnant woman, 42 years old, was asked if the pregnancy was planned at this vulnerable age as her first child was 20 years old. Her response was that she had lost a husband 5 years ago and had recently remarried. She was coping but her challenge was that the first child was rejecting both the new husband and the pregnancy. This was a reflection of another need for psychosocial support that could have been achieved through a proper psychosocial assessment by a midwife and appropriate referral offered.

9. Why should psychosocial risks be screened during antenatal care?

The concept of psychosocial stressors during pregnancy encompasses life experiences, including among others, changes in personal life, job status, family makeup, housing and domestic violence [1]. All these require adaptive coping mechanisms on the part of the pregnant woman, which can be achieved through the support of the midwife.

Risk screening, according to Refs. [1, 7], involves using a list of risk factors and some form of scoring system to classify pregnant women into specific risk categories, typically high risk or low risk, using cutoff points or thresholds. The focus of risk screening is to detect early symptoms and to predict the likelihood of complications. The intention of risk assessment is to predict problems before they occur and, as such, take appropriate action by providing optimal maternal care.

Bibring (1959) as cited by Stahl and Hundley [16] was among the first psychoanalytic writers to claim that "pregnancy is a psychobiological crisis affecting all expectant mothers, no matter what their state of psychic health is. As [with] every normal crisis that constitutes a turning point in life, it precipitates an acute disequilibrium…may lead to a new level of psychological maturity and integration. The outcome of this crisis might have a profound effect not only on the woman herself but also on the mother-child relationship".

A cross-sectional study to identify a relationship between life stress, perceived social support and symptoms of depression and anxiety was conducted by Waldenstrom [34]. Based on her findings, it was recommended that psychosocial assessment of pregnant women and their partners may facilitate interventions to augment support networks and as such reduce the risk of psychosocial stress.

The New Antenatal Care Model proposed by WHO [35] recommends a set of activities during each visit for those women who are identified to be at low risk by screening for conditions likely to increase adverse outcomes of pregnancy, providing therapeutic intervention known to be beneficial and educating women about safe birth. However, the model does not emphasise psychosocial issues but proposes that some time should be set aside during each visit to discuss the pregnancy and related issues. Emphasis was put on the importance of communication.

As a measure to promote psychosocial risk assessment, a new approach to psychosocial risk assessment during pregnancy (ANEW) was implemented in Australia during 2000, in a form of a project to provide an alternative way to psychological risk screening in pregnancy. A training programme in advanced communication skills and common psychosocial aspects of childbirth was offered to midwives and doctors at the Mercy Hospital for women, with the aim of improving the identification and support of women with psychosocial needs in pregnancy [36]. The outcome of the programme was that it improved the ability of the health care professionals to identify and care for women with psychosocial needs.

A randomised controlled trial examining the effectiveness of the Antenatal Psychosocial Health Assessment (ALPHA) form in detecting psychosocial risk factors in pregnant women revealed that 72.7% of the women in the ALPHA group showed interest in discussing psychosocial issues The experimental group was twice as likely to declare psychosocial problems as the control group (based on odds ratio 1.8, 95% confidence interval and 1.1–3.0, $\rho = 0.02$).

Two-thirds of health care providers in the ALPHA group found the form easy to use, and 86% said they would use it if it were recommended as standard practice. The conclusion of the trial showed that the assessment of psychosocial well-being during antenatal care was acceptable to both women and health care professionals [4, 31] in a project on antenatal psychosocial risk assessment in Australia, stating that antenatal depression, domestic violence and postnatal depression occurred more frequently than gestational diabetes, placenta praevia, pre-eclampsia and other obstetric and medical conditions, but most midwifery care settings still do not routinely screen for psychosocial problems.

As stated in Ref. [5] and other literature, for example, Hall (2001) as cited in Ref. [5], the procedures that are commonly undertaken to monitor pregnancy are aimed at reducing morbidity and mortality, but have been found to often cause physical, social and emotional harm. The physiological care that is routinely offered during antenatal care clearly illustrates that the scope of antenatal care is primarily derived from a medical perspective. The implication is that routine antenatal care fails to meet reasonable expectations and the needs of women.

Midwives are urged to overcome the perception in literature and media that health care providers are unkind, rude, unsympathetic and uncaring, as negative emotions such as anger may arise when a woman receives insensitive care. Delwo [37] concluded her study of Swedish women's satisfaction with medical and emotional aspects of antenatal care by urging midwives working in antenatal care to support pregnant women and their partners in a professional and friendly way in order to increase their satisfaction with care. They also advised that identifying and responding to women who are dissatisfied with their antenatal care could help to improve their satisfaction.

10. A study on psychosocial risk assessment and support during pregnancy conducted in Gauteng Province, South Africa

The aim of this study was to develop guidelines for the enhancement of psychosocial risk assessment of pregnant women, with a focus on the provision of psychosocial support.

It was hoped that the results of the study would provide evidence that could motivate interventions aimed at closing the gap between the routine assessment of physiological risks factors and the assessment of psychosocial risk factors during antenatal care. This would provide a basis for midwives to implement an appropriate action should any psychosocial risk be identified. Once formally tested, such guidelines could be incorporated into national guidelines for best practice.

10.1. Ethical considerations

Ethical clearance was obtained from the University of the Witwatersrand Human Research Ethics Committee, protocol number M081013. Participation was voluntary. Anonymity and confidentiality were maintained throughout the research process. The ethical principles of autonomy, beneficence, non-maleficence and justice were observed accordingly.

10.2. Research context and methods

A mixed-method research was used for this study. A sequential explanatory design was employed, whereby quantitative data were first collected and analysed, followed by qualitative data collection and analysis in two consecutive phases [38]. The investigation was conducted within the following contexts:

10.3. Sampling and data collection

Sampling was purposive for all data sources, which were midwifery education and training regulations from the South African Nursing Council; midwifery education and training records of the three nursing colleges providing basic nurse education in Gauteng Province in South Africa; records of antenatal care for women attending government antenatal facilities in Gauteng Province were reviewed to establish the inclusion of psychosocial care; the administration of questionnaires to pregnant women attending antenatal care in Gauteng Province clinics; focus group discussions with both midwives and pregnant women at the antenatal care clinics; a survey to establish the extent of psychosocial assessment and psychosocial care by midwives during pregnancy, through a self-administered questionnaire; and in-depth interviews conducted with midwifery experts from various settings at which midwifery was offered, for example, universities, nursing colleges and midwifery obstetric units (MOUs).

10.4. Data analysis

10.4.1. Quantitative data analysis

Quantitative data were analysed using Stata Release 10 statistical software. Data analysis generally included summary statistics (mean, standard deviation for continuous variables, frequencies and percentages for discrete variables) and Cronbach's alpha for internal consistency. Confidence intervals of 95% were used to report for discrete variable.

10.4.2. Qualitative data analysis

Qualitative data analysis occurred concurrently with data collection. To enhance the depth of qualitative analysis, multiple approaches to data analysis were used (e.g., constant comparison, thematic analysis and framework analysis) comparing themes and categories as a form of across-case analysis technique [38]. The stages that were involved in reducing data were examining, categorising and tabulating data [39].

Data analysis was systematic, sequential, verifiable and continuous in order to minimise potential bias. A "Framework Analysis" was mostly used in qualitative data analysis.

10.5. An overview of study findings and discussion

10.5.1. Quantitative results

The findings confirmed that women experience stressful life events during pregnancy as illustrated in **Table 1**.

The response from 300 participants was that 184 (61.3%) were experiencing stressful life events during the current pregnancy, whereas 116 (38.6%) did not experience any stressful life events. Among those who experienced stressful life events, 72 (24%) experienced two events and 44 (14%) experienced three or more stressful life events. This provides evidence of the importance of assessing women psychosocially as almost all women present with psychosocial problems.

The SANC Regulations, the curriculum and learning guides display a broad approach to psychosocial care as the focus is on holistic care. Written tests, examinations and clinical tools implemented at the colleges address psychosocial care to a minimal level. The Gauteng antenatal care guideline policy, the Guidelines for Maternity Care in South Africa (2015) and the midwifery competency register do not reflect psychosocial content in their guidelines or psychosocial criteria to be met during antenatal care. The antenatal card does not reflect guidelines on psychosocial care, as midwives recorded what they perceived as relevant to be assessed psychosocially.

Pregnancy stressful life events	Women's responses n (%)	
	Yes	No
1.1. Have you experienced death of a spouse or family member?	82(27)	218(73)
1.2. Have you gone through a divorce or marital separation?	26(9)	274(91)
1.3. Were you retrenched or fired from work?	37(12)	264(88)
1.4. Have you been a victim of rape or sexual assault?	15(5)	286(95)
1.5. Have you ever experienced any pregnancy loss?	60(20)	242(80)
2. Was the pregnancy planned?	140(46)	162(54)
3. Have you been sick during this pregnancy?	141(47)	160(53)
If yes, what was the illness?	Note response to the questions below	
4. Have you ever attempted suicide?	15(5)	285(95)
5. Have you ever been diagnosed with a mental health condition?	14(5)	286(95)
6. Have you been hospitalised for a mental health problem?	16(5)	284(95)
7. Did you attend any mental health counselling session?	27(9)	274(91)

Table 1. Stressful life events experienced by respondents during the current.

10.5.2. Qualitative findings

The findings from the focus group discussions within this study also indicated that psychosocial assessment and care were important during pregnancy. The respondents further highlighted the importance of an appropriate guideline and a record for psychosocial assessment and care as reflected within the following responses:

Respondent 1: *"If you look now the state of affairs of our antenatal card it just says social…(***emphasizing***), and you can ask anything… there is nowhere psychosocial issues are recorded".*

Respondent 2: *"Yes, something like TICK, TICK, will help maybe something like a checklist to ask relevant questions, with a checklist I think we would be made aware of the things that we normally don't ask".*

*"Yes, (***All participants***) the checklist will remind us to go deeper, you know beyond the surface, to go deeper than the care that we normally give because it's useless to pretend as if everything is fine whereas the patient has a big problem that can lead to complications, but once we have something that will guide us to ask something, even if you don't ask all the questions, but you know maybe you can highlight, and maybe you pick up something, that will be very helpful".*

Respondent 3: *"There must be a tool because on the green card is just a small line, where we ask for example, it is not written clear, just says "social"… therefore if there was a guideline regarding what should be done it will be appropriate for the pregnant women".*

The concern about the need for training and support for midwives and other health professionals undertaking care to pregnant women [40] led to the development of a psychosocial risk assessment tool that was also based on the findings of the study. Furthermore, there are few studies worldwide reporting the development, evaluation and implementation of screening tools for psychosocial risk factors in pregnant women and subsequent intervention and prevention programs [45]. The assessment tool developed from the findings of this study is currently being piloted in 21 Community Health Centers in Gauteng Province as a 3-year project (2017–2019). The aim of the pilot study is to evaluate the tool, modify it and incorporate it as part of routine antenatal care. The long-term plan is to have a policy developed that integrates psychosocial risk assessment and support with routine physical care.

Based on the increasing international move to standardise as routine the psychosocial assessment and depression screening of all pregnant women and offer relevant support [40–42], different options need to be considered in order to enhance psychosocial care. Some of the interventions that are applied in certain countries globally are reflected in **Table 2**.

10.6. Group antenatal care

Based on the shortage of midwives or clinicians reported in this and other studies, and coupled with a limitation in psychosocial care, group antenatal care might be another option.

Group antenatal care originated a decade ago in Minnesota, USA, during the early 1970s. It was introduced in Denmark in 1998, followed by Sweden in 2000. It is offered concurrently with traditional antenatal care. Antenatal visits are carried out in groups of 6–8. There is evidence that this approach increases networking between pregnant women, women are

Type of intervention	Description
Group antenatal care (Centering Pregnancy, USA)	Consist of a group facilitated by the clinician that lasts approximately 90–120 minutes. This allows a discussion of a wide range of pregnancy-related issues that include psychosocial issues [43].
Hawaiian-style "Talkstory"	The talk-story is integrated into the woman's antenatal and postnatal assessment and care and involves an exchange of thoughts between the woman and midwife. It is based on the woman's values, beliefs and experiences, acknowledging custom and culture.
A psychosocial risk assessment model (PRAM) Australia	Offers a conceptual framework, measures and methods suitable for a brief psychosocial assessment of pregnant and postpartum women [44].
ALPHA tool (Canada)	35 items used to detect 15 risk factors for postnatal adverse psychosocial outcomes [31].
KINDEX (University of Konstanz, Germany)	Assess 11 risk arears during pregnancy, the presence of psychosocial factors and the experience of adversities by women [45]. Has been applied in European countries.
Antenatal risk questionnaire (ANQR)	Composed of 12 items retrieved from the original 23 pregnancy risks [46].

Table 2. Interventions to enhance psychosocial care.

able to validate and sort information within the group and it also allows a midwife to devote more time to pregnant women by saving about 3 hours per woman [47]. Groups may address common psychosocial problems, and those who need further individual consultation can be offered the same, which will probably not be often, with routine individualised care.

The Schindler-Rising model of "centering pregnancy", one of the recommended models for antenatal care, is presented in **Figure 1**.

A "Centering pregnancy" model is an innovative model for prenatal care. It focuses on "woman-centered care" by integrating antenatal care, health information and group support. It acknowledges a woman as an expert regarding her needs. The approach is practised, for example, in Canada, where women are involved in their basic assessment by weighing one another, checking ones' own urine sample, and intragroup checking of blood pressure. Each woman also records results in her own antenatal card [47]

Figure 1. "Centering pregnancy".

A "centering pregnancy" model is an innovative model for prenatal care. It focuses on "woman-centred care" by integrating antenatal care, health information and group support. It acknowledges a woman as an expert regarding her needs. The approach is practised, for example, in Canada, where women are involved in their basic assessment by weighing one another, checking one's own urine sample, and intragroup checking of blood pressure. Each woman also records results in her own antenatal card [47].

Although the "centering pregnancy" model might free midwives or clinicians from routine investigations and as such allow them more time to address issues like psychosocial care, it carries a limitation in a sense that women should be literate, and the process should still be supervised by a midwife or a clinician until women are familiar with all aspects.

10.7. The Hawaiian-style "talkstory"

A Hawaiian-style "talkstory" originated from a needs-assessment project undertaken in Hawaii during 2000, where women indicated that their psychosocial needs were largely unmet.

A Hawaiian-style "talkstory" could offer an ideal approach in offering culturally focused antenatal care as it is a culturally based interactive communication approach, aimed at addressing the pregnant woman's psychosocial needs. It could be mostly effective during the initial antenatal care booking as the woman is taking the lead in sharing her childbirth experiences. **Figure 2** explains the talkstory process as a guideline for midwives who might be interested in its implementation.

"talkstory process"

The "talkstory" process involves a pregnant woman taking the lead in sharing her experiences and expectations with a midwife or a clinician in her care, as a form of assessment. The woman is given an opportunity to articulate what she feels is important for her pregnancy and if there are problems. Her suggestions as to how to overcome the problems are sought. The interpretation of data obtained during the discussion is determined between the woman and the midwife.

Figure 2. The "talkstory" process.

http://dx.doi.org/10.5772/intechopen.80394

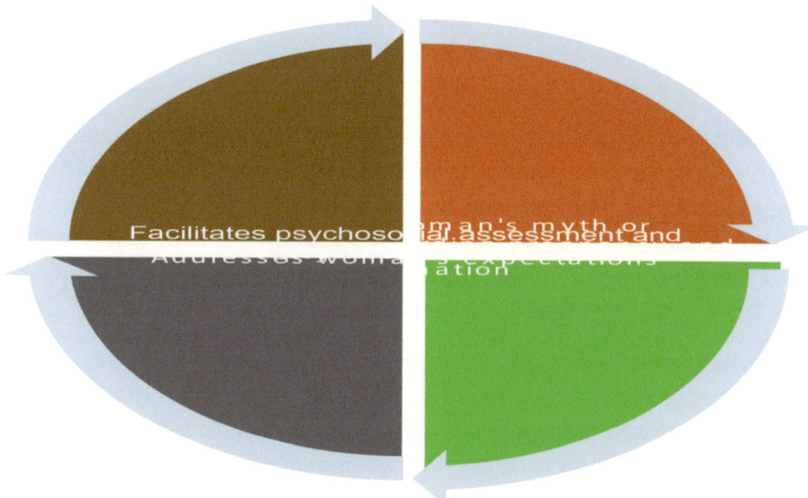

Figure 3. Outcomes achieved through the "talkstory process".

10.8. The success of the "talkstory" approach

The "talkstory" approach, as illustrated in **Figure 3**, served as an ideal way of assessing women psychosocially. It offers an opportunity to provide the woman with relevant health information and to validate myths or misconceptions about childbirth that the woman might be having, while also addressing her expectations. This is a type of psychosocial assessment and care that is women-centred, through placing an emphasis on a woman's own beliefs, offering her autonomy and a right to informed choice [48].

A "talkstory" is an ideal approach during the initial contact of the woman and the midwife or a clinician, and as such it might promote communication between the two; it needs some time and requires a midwife or clinician who is skilled in listening and who has an ability to convey compassion, acceptance and encouragement to the woman. This approach might be a challenge in institutions experiencing the shortage of staff.

The implementation of psychosocial care incorporates adherence to the following principles: human rights and equality, justice and confidentiality. Measures to be put in place as part of psychosocial support are availability of referral resources (social, mental, economic and judicial); the assessor should be well informed about the options of referral and to consider the possibility of the accompaniment of the woman throughout the process as a form of continuity of care and as stated by the United Nations Entity for Gender Equality and the Empowerment of Women.

11. Conclusion

The issue of psychosocial risk assessment and support seems to be a concern both nationally and internationally. The process of adapting to pregnancy and the resulting life changes are often difficult, even if the pregnancy is planned as pregnancy involves intense emotional, spiritual, psychological and social factors that need a midwife's caring awareness and responsiveness.

A pregnant woman should be assisted to recognise and incorporate these changes into her self-image, her social network and her lifestyle. When the pregnancy is unplanned, the psychosocial changes may be more profound and lead to uncertainty, anxiety and depression [19].

There is a growing need for understanding the place and significance of maternal psychology and other psychosocial factors in the management of pregnant women by midwives or clinicians. Strategies for supporting maternal and foetal mental health need to be developed, as the importance of a good-quality pregnancy extends beyond antenatal care. Psychosocial risk assessment during pregnancy is further considered as the first strategy to support maternal well-being as this will allow the pregnant woman to cope with her pregnancy [26].

In theory, risk assessment is a logical tool for rationalising service delivery to ensure that those in greater need receive special attention and care. However, it is becoming increasingly clear that with incorrect and inadequate psychosocial risk assessment, scarce resources may be diverted away from pregnant women who are in real need. However, in the absence of evidence of an effective risk screening process, risk assessment cannot be relied on as a basis for matching needs and care in maternity services [7]. Ideally, psychosocial risk assessment should be included within the overall risk assessment or could be administered as a separate tool in the form of a checklist.

Author details

Johanna Mmabojalwa Mathibe-Neke[1]* and Seipati Suzan Masitenyane[2]

*Address all correspondence to: mathijm@unisa.ac.za

1 University of South Africa, Pretoria, South Africa

2 Medicure Clinic, Gauteng Province, South Africa

References

[1] Chitra L, Gnanadurai A. Psychosocial outcomes of pregnancy in women living with HIV in Coimbatore district of Tamil Nadu. Journal of Dental and Medical Sciences. 2015; **14**(1):120-125

[2] World Health Organisation. Safe Motherhood: Every Pregnancy Faces a risk. Geneva: Switzerland; 1998

[3] Kaaya SF, Mbwambo JK, Kilonzo GP, Van Den Borne H, Leshabari MT, Smith Fawzi MC, et al. Socio-economic and partner relationship factors associated with antenatal depressive morbidity among pregnant women in Dar es Salaam, Tanzania. Tanzania Journal of Health Research. 2010;**12**(1):1-15

[4] Pereira PK, Lovisi GM, Pilowsky DL, Lima LA, Legay LF. Depression during pregnancy: Prevalence and risk factors among women attending a public health clinic in Rio de Janeiro, Brazil. Cadernos de Saúde Pública. 2009;**25**(12):2725-2736

[5] Willinck L, Schubert R. Antenatal psychosocial risk assessment project. Australian College of Midwives Incorporated. 2000:7-12

[6] Clinical Guideline 2003. Antenatal Care Routine Care for the Healthy Pregnant Woman. London: National Collaborating Centre for Women's and Children's Health Commissioned by the National Institute for Clinical Excellence: Royal College of Obstetricians and Gynecologists Press; 2003. pp. 26-40

[7] Baldo MH. The antenatal care debate. Review. Eastern Mediterranean Health Journal. 2001;**7**(6):1046-1055

[8] Mehdizadeh A, Roosta F, Chaichian S, Alaghehbandan R. Evaluation of the impact of birth preparation courses on the health of the mother and the newborn. American Journal of Perinatology. 2005;**22**(1):7-9

[9] O'Keane V, Marsh MS. Depression during pregnancy. British Medical Journal. 2007; **334**(7601):1003-1005

[10] Dodd JM, Robinson SJ, Crowther AC. Guiding antenatal care. The Medical Journal of Australia. 2002;**176**(6):253-254

[11] Gelder MG, Lo'pez-Ibor J, Anderson NC. New Oxford Textbook of Psychiatry. Vol. 2. Oxford: Oxford University Press; 2003. 2131 p

[12] Goodman JH. Womens' mental health. Journal of Obstetric Gynecology and Neonatal Nursing. 2005;**34**:245 Medline

[13] Handley MC. Emotional responses to pregnancy based on geographical classification of residence. Online Journal of Rural Nursing and Health Care. 2006;**6**(2):7-1

[14] Woodward V. Caring for women: The potential contribution of formal theory to midwifery practice. Midwifery. 2000;**16**:68-75

[15] Parry DC. We wanted a birth experience, not a medical experience: Exploring Canadian women's use of midwifery. Health Care for Women International. 2008;**29**(8):784-806

[16] Stahl K, Hundley V. Risk and risk assessment in pregnancy: Do we scare because we care? Midwifery. 2003;**19**(4):298-309

[17] Dejin-Karlsson E, Ostergon PO. Psychosocial factors, lifestyle and foetal growth: the added value of of both pre- and post-natal. The European Journal of Public Health. 2003; **13**(3):210-217

[18] Hollander D. Poor psychosocial support raises the odds of having an underweight infant. Guttmacher Digest: Family Planning Perspectives. 2000;**32**(3):1-3

[19] Langer A. Support During Pregnancy for Women at an Increased Risk of Low Birthweight Babies: RHL Commentary. The WHO Reproductive Library; Geneva: World Health Organisation; 2003. pp. 1-2

[20] Namagembe I. Prevalence of Stress, Depression, Alcohol Use, and Social Support among HIV Infected and Uninfected Pregnant Women in Uganda. Washington, DC: APHA Annual Meeting and Expo; 2007

[21] Coussons-Read ME, Okun ML, Nettles CD. Psychosocial stress increases inflammatory markers and alters cytokine production across pregnancy. Brain Behavior and Immunty. 2007;**21**(3):343-350

[22] Rondo PHC, Ferreira RF, Nogueira F, Lobert H, Artes R. Marternal psychological stress and distress as predictors of low birth weight, prematurity and intrauterine growth retardation. European Journal of Clinical Nutrition. 2002;**57**:266-272

[23] Raynor M, Sullivan A, Oates M. Why mothers die: A public health concern. British Journal of Midwifery. 2003;**11**(6):393-395

[24] Matthey S. Assessing for psychosocial morbidity in pregnant women. Canadian Medical Association Journal. 2005;**173**(3):267-269

[25] Hamid F, Asif A, Haider II. Study of anxiety and depression during pregnancy. Pakistan Journal of Medical Sciences. 2008;**24**(6):861-864

[26] Shamim ul Moula SM. Health care behaviour: Factors influencing health care behaviour of a person [PhD thesis]. Blog Archive. 2009. Available from: http://ealthcarebehavior-shamim.blogspot.com/2009/06/psychosocial-factors-related-t [Accessed: May 12, 2011]

[27] Smith MV, Brunetto WL, Yonkers KA. Identifying perinatal depression-sooner is better. Contemporary Obstetric and Gynecology. 2004;**49**:58

[28] Glazier RH, Elgar FJ, Goel V, Holzapfel S. Stress, social support and emotional distress in a community sample of pregnant women. Journal of Psychosomatic Obstetrics and Gynaecology. 2004;**25**(3-4):247-255

[29] Fawole AO, Okunlola MA, Adekunle AO. Client's perceptions of the quality of antenatal care. Journal of the National Medical Association. 2008;**100**(9):1052-1057

[30] Gunn J, Hegarty K, Nagle C, Forster D, Brown S, Lumley J. Putting women-centered care into practice: A new approach to psychosocial risk assessment during pregnancy (ANEW). Birth. 2006;**33**(1):46-55

[31] Carroll JC, Reid AJ, Biringer A, Midmer D, Glazier RH, Wilson L, et al. Effectiveness of the antenatal psychosocial health assessment (ALPHA) form in detecting psychosocial concerns: Arandomised controlled trial. Canadian Medical Association Journal. 2005;**73**(3): 253-259. DOI: 10.1503/cmaj.1040610

[32] Hildingsson I, Radestad I. Sweddish women's satisfaction with medical and emotional aspects of antenatal care. Journal of Advanced Nursing. 2005;**52**(3):239-249

[33] Suppaseemanont W. Depression in pregnancy: Drug safety and nursing management. The American Journal of Maternal Child Nursing. 2006;**31**(1):10-15

[34] Waldenstrom U. Why do some women change their opinion about childbirth over time? Birth. 2004;**31**(2):102-107

[35] Feldman P. Social support during pregnancy can affect foetal growth and birthweight. Psychosomatic Medicine. Journal of the American Psychosomatic Society. 2000. Available from: http://www.cfah.org/hbns/newsrelease/social9-22-00.cfm [Accessed: Jul 7, 2007]

[36] Seimyr L, Edhborg M, Lundh W, Sjogren B. In the shadow of maternal depression mood: Experiences of parenthood during the first year after birth. Journal of Psychosomatic Obstetrics and Gynaecology. 2004;**25**(1):23-34

[37] Delwo K. Women's Health Issues—Feminist Medicine. 2010. Available from: http://www.suite101.com/content/womens-health-issues---feminist-medicine-a320107

[38] Christensen LB, Johnson RB, Turner LA. Research Methods, Design, and Analysis. 12th ed. Edingburg Gate, England: Pearson Education limited; 2015. p. 542

[39] Rabiee F. Focus group interview and data analysis. Proceedings of the Nutrition Society. 2004;**63**:655-660

[40] Rollans M, Schmied V, Meade T. We just ask some questions… the process of antenatal psychosocialassessment by midwives. Midwifery. 2013;**29**:935-942

[41] Kalra H, Reilly N, Austin M. An evaluation of routine antenatal depression screening and psychosocial assessment in a regional private maternity setting in Australia. Journal of Obstetric and Gynaecology. 2018:1-14

[42] Castillo-Torralba M. Psychosocial and Psychological Interventions for Preventing Postpartum Depression: RHL Commentary. The WHO Reproductive Health Library, Geneva: World Health Organisation; 2008. pp. 1-5

[43] Novick G, Reid AE, Lewis J, Kershaw TS, Schindler Rising S, Ickovics JR. Group prenatal care: model fidelity and outcomes. American Journal of Obstetric and Gynecology. 2013; **112**:1-6

[44] Priest SR, Austin MP, Barnett BB, Buist A. A psychosocial risk assessment model (PRAM) for use with pregnant and postpartum women in primary care settings. Archives of Women's Mental Health. 2008;**11**:307-317

[45] Spyridou A, Schauer M, Ruf-Leushner M. Obstetric care providers assessing psychosocial risk factors during pregnancy: Validation of a short screening tool—KINDEX Spanish Version. Child and Adolescent Psychiatry and Mental Health. 2014;**8**(30):1-15

[46] Austin M, Colton J, Priest S, Reilly N, Hadzi-Pavlovic D. The antenatal risk questionnaire (ANRQ): Acceptability and use for psychosocial risk assessment in the maternity setting. Women and Birth. 2013;**26**(1):17-25

[47] Wedin K, Molin J, Crang Svalenius EL. Group antenatal care: New pedagogic method for antenatal care—A pilot study. 2010

[48] Poat A, McElligott M, Fleming V. How midwives attitudes can affect the research process. British Journal of Midwifery. 2003;**11**(6):396-400

Chapter 3

Pregnancy Weight Gain: The Short Term and the Long Term

Ruth Mielke

Additional information is available at the end of the chapter

http://dx.doi.org/10.5772/intechopen.79066

Abstract

Achieving adequate pregnancy weight gain is critical to optimize infant and maternal outcomes. Extremes of pregnancy weight gain—excessive and inadequate—can jeopardize the health of the mother and her baby. Excessive pregnancy weight gain is associated with increased risk of pregnancy complications, cesarean delivery, and an overly large infant. In the longer term, women with excessive gain during pregnancy are prone to retain pregnancy weight and are at risk for life-long obesity and diabetes. Inadequate gain is associated with negative infant outcomes such as low birth weight, growth restriction, and increased risk for cardiovascular disease as an adult. Worldwide, more women are entering pregnancy overweight or obese. This trend is a more recent phenomenon even in developing countries. Some countries or regions have guidelines for pregnancy weight gain but others do not. The 2009 United States Institute of Medicine Guidelines are presented and discussed for the general population or women during pregnancy as well as for less clear-cut cases, such as twins and women with extreme obesity. Midwives and health workers need to be comfortable discussing guidelines for pregnancy weight gain in their settings—whether in a classroom, home, or clinic.

Keywords: pregnancy weight gain, gestational weight gain, postpartum weight retention, prepregnancy body mass index, postpartum weight retention

1. Introduction

Achieving adequate pregnancy weight gain (PWG) is critical to optimize infant and maternal outcomes [1]. In developed countries, excessive pregnancy weight gain (PWG) is more likely [2–6] while women in lower-resource countries are more likely to experience inadequate PWG [7–9]. Inadequate PWG is mainly associated with poorer infant outcomes, preterm birth, suboptimal infant birth weight [10–12], and greater risk of infant death [13]. Excessive PWG is also associated with negative infant outcomes (e.g., excessive infant birth weights [11, 14]), but in mothers, it increases the likelihood of delivery complications including cesarean delivery [14–16], postpartum weight retention [11, 17], and subsequent obesity [18–20]. In the longer term, inadequate and excessive PWG appear to alter the fetal intrauterine environment, resulting in obesity in childhood [21–23], adolescence [24, 25], and type 2 diabetes, and atherogenic profiles in adulthood [26, 27]. Therefore, optimizing PWG improves not only maternal health but that of the next generation.

2. Pregnancy weight gain: physiology and composition

Pregnancy boasts an astounding array of physiologic and developmental changes that support the fetus from conception to birth. Physiologic changes include those necessary for fetal sustenance and growth; adequate oxygenation of the maternal/fetal dyad during pregnancy; and future provision for newborn nutrition via lactation after delivery. Throughout pregnancy, the mother's metabolism adjusts based on hormonal changes of pregnancy, fetal requirements, her nutritional intake, and her level of physical activity. These changes are reflected in pregnancy weight gain (PWG), which includes gains in maternal and fetal fat mass and fat-free mass (protein, skeletal tissue), as well as the placenta and amniotic fluid [1, 28]. A complete review of pregnancy physiology is beyond the scope of this chapter. However, it is important for midwives and health-care workers to understand how aspects of pregnancy physiology affect PWG.

The appearance of pregnancy-associated hormones and concurrent increases in existing hormones have multi-factorial influences on PWG. Referred to as the hormone of pregnancy, human chorionic gonadotropin (hCG) can be detected within days of embryo implantation. Serum concentrations of hCG rise steeply and peak about 60 days after conception—about 7 weeks after the first day of the last menstrual period (LMP) [29].

The dramatic surge of hCG in early pregnancy along with increases in other maternal hormones such as estrogen and progesterone are believed to contribute to the common experience of "morning sickness" which often starts at the fifth week after the last menstrual period (LMP), peaks at 8–12 weeks, and resolves by 16–18 weeks in only a small number of women in whom the symptoms persist past 20 weeks of gestation. Such vomiting (emesis) can result in small weight loss in the first half of pregnancy. As long as the mother is not dehydrated and has not lost more than 5% of her initial body weight, non-pharmacologic relief measures should be offered and she can be reassured that hyperemesis will not negatively impact the pregnancy outcome if her pregnancy weight gain normalizes. Such measures include ginger, chamomile, vitamin B6, and/or acupuncture [30]. One study showed that nausea and vomiting in pregnancy minimized the risk of excessive PWG, particularly in women with high prepregnancy body mass indices (BMIs) [31]. However, if the mother has severe nausea and vomiting (hyperemesis gravidarum) resulting in electrolyte imbalance, dehydration, and weight loss greater than 5% of her prepregnancy weight, she will require medical treatment inclusive of intravenous fluids [32]. Severe nausea may also be a sign of other illnesses, such as gastroenteritis (stomach bugs), migraines, or gallbladder or pancreas disease [33].

Within a week of conception, the placenta begins to secrete another new hormone, human placental lactogen (hPL), thought to influence several metabolic processes associated with PWG. hPL blunts maternal insulin actions to ensure that sufficient protein and other energy sources are available to the fetus. The rate of HPL secretion parallels placental growth resulting in increasing insulin resistance making increased nutrition available to the fetus as the pregnancy progresses. In addition, hPL promotes maternal lipolysis which increases the circulating levels of free fatty acids to accommodate fetal nutritional and maternal metabolic needs [33, 34]. If a lipid panel (cholesterol, triglycerides, and other lipid fractions) is done for some reason during pregnancy, midwives and health-care workers should expect that levels will be elevated. This is evidence of the increased availability of energy being made available to the fetus during pregnancy!

Increased levels of progesterone and estrogen, both steroid hormones, contribute and respond to changes in PWG. Both hormones are initially synthesized by the corpus luteum of the ovary until about 7–9 gestational weeks when a "luteal-placental" shift occurs and the placenta takes over their production [35]. Increased hormone levels of estrogen influence carbohydrate, lipid, and bone metabolism [29] and promote growth of the uterus and breast tissue. High levels of progesterone ("pro-gestation") maintain the pregnancy by keeping the distended uterus in a quiescent state and suppress the mother's immune response to the fetus so that it is not rejected. Progesterone and estrogen contribute to the decrease in maternal vascular resistance to accommodate the notable increase (40–50% above her baseline) of maternal blood volume for better transit of nutrients and oxygen [33, 35]. Increased maternal blood volume contributes to PWG as does increased extracellular volume (edema).

Pyrosis (heartburn) affects 50–80% of women in late pregnancy. It occurs when progesterone relaxes the lower esophageal sphincter (opening) and a burning sensation occurs as the acidic content of the mother's stomach irritates the esophagus [33]. In some cultures it is believed that mothers with heartburn in pregnancy will have infants with thick heads of hair! Nonpharmacologic approaches for women with heartburn include advice to eat smaller, more frequent meals, avoid trigger foods (e.g., high in fat or spicy foods), and avoid eating too close to bedtime or at times that they plan to be recumbent. The first-line pharmacologic approach is oral antacids containing cations of sodium bicarbonate (baking soda), calcium carbonate (TUMS), or magnesium salts which are widely available in stores and clinics. Antacids that contain calcium or magnesium are recommended as calcium is often needed and magnesium may reduce the incidence of preeclampsia [36]. If these do not work, women may also be given more targeted agents like H2 receptor agonists (cimetidine or ranitidine) or proton-pump inhibitors (omeprazole) by their midwife or clinic [33, 36]. Although no woman wants to experience heartburn in pregnancy, she can be reassured that it may stimulate more healthy eating behaviors and therefore may limit the possibility of excessive PWG.

Pregnancy is a teachable moment in which women are more likely to adopt risk-reducing behaviors and to pursue learning about their health and its effects on the growth and development of the fetus [37–39]. Midwives and other health-care workers are well positioned to provide accurate advice and counseling on PWG that can positively impact the outcome of the pregnancy. In a study of Hispanic women in Los Angeles, 18.8% of the women did not recall any discussions about PWG with health-care providers during pregnancy. Among those who had such discussions, only 42% reported receiving weight gain advice within the Institute of Medicine (IOM) guidelines [1], 16.5% below guidelines, and 10% above. The other women (13.5%) who reported having the discussion did not recall the recommended weight gain amount. Compared with women who received accurate advice on PWG, women who reported advice below IOM guidelines were 1.7 times more likely to gain less than the recommended amount and those who reported advice above IOM guidelines were 2.0 times more likely to gain excessive PWG [40]. This demonstrates that (1) health-care workers must be knowledgeable on PWG recommendations, (2) accurate PWG information should be a routine part of pregnancy care, and (3) when accurate advice is given, women are more likely to gain appropriately during pregnancy.

2.1. Composition of pregnancy weight gain

Pregnancy weight gain is the sum of maternal, placental, and fetal components. Over the course of pregnancy, protein, fat, water, and minerals are deposited in the fetus, placenta, amniotic fluid, uterus, mammary gland (breasts), blood, and adipose (fat) tissue. The products of conception (placenta, fetus, amniotic fluid) comprise approximately one-third of the total pregnancy weight gain [28] (**Table 1**).

2.1.1. Body water

Total body water accumulation is highly variable during pregnancy. Healthy women accumulate an additional 7–8 L of water which is distributed in the fetus (32%), blood (17%), amniotic fluid (10%), uterus (10%), breasts (4%), and in women with no edema or just mild leg swelling (20%) throughout the maternal tissues. Visible leg edema or noted changes like rings being too tight occur in 50–85% of women during pregnancy. However, some women accumulate much more water by the end of pregnancy. This can be as much as more than 3–4 L over typical water accumulation. Overweight women have greater generalized edema than underweight women [28] as do some women with hypertensive disorders (chronic/gestational hypertension and preeclampsia) during pregnancy. Previous definitions of preeclampsia included excessive edema in the diagnosis [41] but this is not current practice [42]. In of itself, excessive edema can be uncomfortable and unsightly, but in the absence of complications, it does not warrant the use of a diuretic (water pill).

2.1.2. Protein

The normally nourished body has little capacity to store protein [28]. Therefore, additional protein accumulated occurs predominantly in late pregnancy when the fetal needs are greatest [29]. In contrast to water accumulation, which is mostly maternal during pregnancy, protein is accumulated predominantly in the fetus (42%) and less so in the uterus (17%), blood (14%), placenta (10%), and breasts (8%) [28]. A Cochrane review of studies of protein and energy intake in pregnancy concluded that dietary advice was effective to increase pregnant women's energy and protein intake and that balanced energy/protein supplementation improves fetal growth and therefore may reduce the risk of perinatal death. However, high-protein or balanced-protein supplementation alone was not beneficial and could be harmful to the fetus [43]. Other factors that require increased demand for protein such as infections and mild-to-moderate energy deficits (common in developing countries) should also be appropriately considered in assessing protein and energy needs [44] (Appendix A).

2.1.3. Fat

Fat accumulation in pregnancy supports the production of steroid hormones (estrogen and progesterone) and provides energy for the mother and her baby. Most of the fat accumulated (approximately 3.3 kg) goes to maternal stores, providing an energy reserve of approximately 30,000 kcal. Maternal fat stores are gained primarily between the 10th and 30th weeks of gestation before fetal energy demands are at their peak [29] and are stored more as visceral rather than subcutaneous fat [45]. Women with appropriate access to food during pregnancy will notice that their hips, back, and lower body feel fuller or more rounded, even before there is abdominal evidence of the pregnancy. If the mother gains within recommendations for her prepregnancy BMI, fat accumulation is inversely related to BMI. Therefore, obese women gain significantly less fat than underweight and normal-weight women. However, in the context of excessive gain, this results in additional visceral fat accumulation which portends higher risk of life-long obesity and other co-morbidities.

2.1.4. Placenta

Pregnancy weight gain is influenced not only by changes in maternal physiology and metabolism but also by placental metabolism. When blood flow is persistently reduced on both sides (fetal and maternal) of the placental exchange, growth restriction results due to decreased oxygen and nutrient access by the fetus. In such cases, the placenta mobilizes some nutrients from maternal stores [46]. Conversely, when there is a surplus of nutrients as in the case of maternal diabetes, excessive PWG, or maternal obesity, fetal overgrowth is more likely.

Tissues and fluids	Weight gained (g)	Weight gained (lb)
Fetus	3400	7.5
Placenta	650	1.4
Amniotic fluid	800	1.8
Uterus	970	2.1
Mammary glands	405	0.9
Blood	1450	3.2
No edema or leg edema only	7675	–
Extracellular extravascular fluid	1480	3.3
Maternal fat stores	3345	7.4
Total weight gained (no edema)	**12,500**	**27.6**
Generalized edema	7675	–
Extracellular extravascular fluid	4697	10.4
Maternal fat stores	2128	4.7
Total weight gained (edema)	**14,500**	**32.0**

Source: Adapted from Hyttena and Chamberlain [28]. Table 7.11, Analysis of weight gain; p. 195.

Table 1. Tissues and fluids and weight gained by 40 weeks of gestation.

However, it is unlikely that varying levels of blood flow and nutrients alone are responsible for fetal undergrowth or overgrowth. It has been recently postulated that the placenta has independent nutrient sensor functions [47]. According to this hypothesis the maternal supply of nutrients and oxygen are actively regulated by placental nutrient transporters. Therefore, beyond passive filtering of available maternal substrate, the placenta has an active role up- or down regulating transport proteins according to the maternal environment.

2.1.5. Fetus

As noted previously, the fetus demands most of the later pregnancy maternal intake of protein. The rapid rate of fetal growth during the last half of gestation dictates changes in basal metabolism, protein, and mineral accumulations. About 60% of the increase in mother's basal metabolic rate (BMR) occurs during the last half of gestation, when the fetal tissue synthesis is the greatest [29]. As there is no evidence that pregnant women store protein early in gestation for later fetal demands, the increased requirements of late pregnancy must be met by increased maternal intake.

The term fetus has more body fat than most other mammalian species. At birth the human fetus has approximately 12–16% body fat while laboratory animals may have just 1–2% body fat at birth. After 30 weeks of gestation, a small loss of maternal body fat occurs while fetal fat mass increases. During this period, 94% of all fat deposition in the fetus occurs [46].

2.2. Pregnancy weight gain recommendations

Midwives and other health workers must be familiar with PWG recommendations specific to their region and know how to apply these based on their assessment of the mother's prepregnancy weight category. In the United States, pregnancy weight gain guidelines were first established by the Institute of Medicine in 1990 [48] and were revised in 2009 due to the increasing prevalence of obesity and new knowledge regarding pregnancy [1]. A key change in the revised guidelines was the use of World Health Organization (WHO) body mass index (BMI) categories instead of categories based on tables used by the US-based Metropolitan Life Insurance Company. One significant result of the application of the WHO BMI categories was that fewer women are categorized as underweight prior to pregnancy (**Table 2**). This is important as the prior underweight BMI cut-off (<19.8) inappropriately classified younger adolescents as underweight when their prepregnancy BMI was actually appropriate for their age [49, 50].

Another significant change was the addition of a specific and narrower range of recommended gain for women who are obese at the onset of pregnancy (**Table 3**). **Table 3** presents the application of the WHO BMI categories, recommended PWG, and rates of PWG for second and third trimesters.

In many cultures, mothers are encouraged to "eat for two" starting in early pregnancy. However, for all but very underweight women, the first trimester through the first half of pregnancy does not require greater food intake but should be focused on the avoidance of harmful substances (e.g., alcohol and nicotine) and more attention to the quality of maternal nutrition rather than increasing the quantity of food. Additional energy intake is recommended

BMI category	IOM 1990 (kg/m^2)	IOM 2009 (kg/m^2)
Underweight	<19.8	<18.5
Normal weight	19.8–26	18.5–24.9
Overweight	26.1–29	25–29.9
Obese class I	>29	30–34.9
Obese class II	–	35–39.9

Table 2. Comparison of Institute of Medicine (IOM) and World Health Organization (WHO) BMI categories.

	Total weight Pregnancy weight Gain		Rates of weight gain 2nd and 3rd trimester1	
Prepregnancy BMI (kg/m^2)	Range (kg)	Range (lbs)	Mean (kg/week)	Mean (lb/week)
Underweight <18.5	12.5–18	28–40	0.51	1
Normal 18.5–24.9	11.5–16	25–35	0.42	1
Overweight 25.0–29.9	7–11.5	15–25	0.28	0.6
Obese >30	5–9	11–20	0.22	0.5

Calculations assume a 1.1–4.4 lbs/0.50–2 kg weight gain in the first trimester.
Adapted from Institute of Medicine [47]. Table S-1 New Recommendations for Total and Rate of Weight Gain during Pregnancy, by Prepregnancy BMI.

Table 3. Institute of Medicine recommended weight gains for pregnancy 1.

more so in the second and third trimesters when greater than 90% of fetal growth occurs. Approximately an additional 340 and 450 kcal are recommended during the second and third trimesters, respectively [51]. However, in well-nourished women, optimal weight gain and outcome of pregnancy can be attained over a very wide range of energy intakes. Many women sustain a pregnancy with a successful outcome on less than the recommended energy intake [29]. This probably reflects different adaptive strategies (reduced physical activity, more effective use of nutrients, etc.) that can be used to meet the additional energy demands of pregnancy.

2.2.1. Global considerations

Worldwide, pregnancy weight gain guidelines may differ from the 2009 IOM guidelines or in some cases, countries may not have PWG guidelines. Although adverse effects are associated with extremes of PWG, there are no WHO guidelines at global or European levels, nor consensus on recommended weight gain in obese women [52]. In 2016, WHO European Region Member States (n = 53) were queried to assess whether there were recommendations in place on appropriate PWG. Two-thirds of the countries (36 countries) reported having national recommendations on appropriate pregnancy weight gain; one-fifth (12 countries) did not have PWG recommendations; and five countries did not respond. Of the 36 countries with recommendations, two-thirds reported recommendations based on prepregnancy BMI for singleton pregnancies, with 21 of those countries using WHO BMI categories. Thirteen countries based their recommendations on the 2009 IOM ones, with four of the thirteen countries modifying guidelines based on IOM guidance. Six countries reported not using WHO BMI categories. Furthermore, three countries said they have different recommendations for each obese class [52].

Some countries utilize prenatal weight gain grids/charts to show the mother how much she should gain based on her weight category and her trends of PWG. The Rosso and Mardones chart is used in most Chilean prenatal clinics, attended by the majority of the country's middle- and low-income women. Other Latin American countries, that is, Argentina, Brazil, Ecuador, Panama, and Uruguay, have also been using this weight gain chart in their prenatal care programs [53, 54]. The Rosso and Mardones chart categorizes maternal nutritional status early in pregnancy based on weight/height, expressed either as the percentage of standard weight (PSW) or body mass index (BMI). The chart shows the desired trend of desirable gestational weight gains for each of these categories. Similar style grids are used in publically funded clinics in many areas of the United States [55, 56] (Appendix B). The graphical depiction of maternal nutritional status and trending PWG patterns are useful for workers and patients with varying literacy levels.

2.2.2. *Asian women*

There is increased attention to pregnancy weight gain guidelines that account for ethnic characteristics and population-based differences. For instance, even with typically lower BMIs, many Asian groups have a higher proportion of body fat (more often in the waist area [central obesity]) and therefore have greater risk of type 2 diabetes and cardiovascular disease than European groups. In 2004, WHO experts discussed this issue and recommended lower BMI cut-offs for Asians in that there is a different correlation between BMI, body fat deposition, and health risk than Europeans [57]. The WHO Asian BMI classification (underweight, <18.5; normal weight, 18.5 to <23; overweight, 23 to <27.5; obese, ≥27.5) narrows the range of normal weight and substantially lowers the thresholds for overweight and obese BMI categories, thereby identifying a larger proportion of persons who in actuality are at a higher risk for cardiovascular disease and type 2 diabetes (**Table 3**).

The WHO Asian BMI categories subsequently spurred interest in studying whether there should also be PWG recommendations specific for Asian women [6, 58–61]. Multi-ethnic Asian (Chinese, Malay, Indian) women in Singapore (n = 1529) were studied to assess PWG ranges for optimal infant outcomes (size of infant appropriate for gestational age [AGA] vs. large or small for gestational age [LGA or SGA]) and maternal outcomes (cesarean vs. vaginal delivery). Outcomes for underweight women were best when they gained more weight as per the IOM guidelines (12.9–23.9 kg vs. 12.5–18 kg) and less weight if overweight (2.6–14.0 kg vs. 7–11.5 kg) or obese (−5.0 to 7.0 kg vs. 5–9 kg). Of note, the optimum range for Singaporean women in the obese category suggested that even weight loss during pregnancy was associated with optimum maternal and fetal outcomes.

In this chapter, the IOM 2009 guideline for PWG is used because it is considered to be applicable to various racial and ethnic groups. However, researchers realize that much further study needs to be done as there are body composition characteristics unique to different racial and ethnic groups which many necessitate recommendations specific to certain groups.

2.2.3. *Total pregnancy weight gain*

Total PWG is the amount of weight a woman gains between conception and the onset of labor [1]. Obtaining an accurately measured weight at both conception and the onset of labor can be difficult if the woman was unsure when conception occurred or due to the lack of awareness of her weight prior to pregnancy. Further, discrepancies between weight reported on a home scale as compared to a clinic or hospital scale are well known. Some women may not have a home scale and because of limited access to health facilities may have little idea of their weight.

However, total PWG is best defined as final pregnancy weight minus her prepregnancy weight. Initial weight can be a prepregnancy weight that is (1) reported by the woman, (2) measured in the clinic, (3) identified from the woman's medical charts at the date closest to conception, or (4) measured at the first prenatal/study visit. The determination of the final pregnancy weight can also be problematic. Hospital emergency departments/birth facilities may not routinely weigh women as part of the labor admission process. However, the woman's self-reported weight is more accurate than estimation by the health-care workers and so should be considered [62, 63].

2.2.4. *Body mass index*

Body mass index (BMI) is but one measure of body composition—specifically fat composition. Other methods to assess body fat composition (e.g., skin fold thickness, underwater weighing, magnetic resonance imaging, dual energy X-ray absorptiometry [DEXA], and ultrasound) are less used in pregnancy because they are either not practical, potentially harmful, or confounded by pregnancy changes such as increases in total body water by 5–8 L [28, 64].

At present, BMI is the most commonly used method of assessing body fat composition worldwide. The BMI categories recommended by the WHO indicate degrees of thinness and fatness and in so doing identify individuals and/or populations at risk for cardiovascular disease, type 2 diabetes, and other related health conditions [65]. For policy purposes, BMI categories are applied to population data to inform and initiate policy, to facilitate prevention programs, and to measure the effect of interventions. BMI categories are also used to identify high-risk individuals for screening; identify individuals for absolute risk assessment; determine the type and intensity of treatment; and monitor individuals for effects of treatment over time [57] (**Table 4**).

Midwives and health-care workers must see that accurate assessment of the mother's prepregnancy BMI is a key starting point on the road map to positive perinatal outcomes: a healthy weight-term infant, avoidance of pregnancy complications (hypertension and diabetes), increased likelihood of vaginal delivery, optimization of breastfeeding, and reduction of postpartum weight retention and subsequent life-long obesity.

Determination of the mother's prepregnancy BMI is body mass category based on her height and weight. As discussed earlier, assessment of the woman's prepregnancy weight is determined based on the best available reported or measured weight; e.g., first prenatal visit especially if in first trimester, or most recent clinic weight prior to the pregnancy. There are many BMI calculators that are easily available to midwives and health-care workers. Body mass index is based on a mathematical computation using the woman's height. The formula is $kg/m^2 = BMI$ where kg is a person's weight in kilograms and m^2 is their height in meters squared. This can

Classification	BMI (kg/m^2)	
	Principal cut-off points	**Asian cut-off points**
Underweight	**<18.50**	**<18.50**
Severe thinness	<16.00	<16.00
Moderate thinness	16.00–16.99	16.00–16.99
Mild thinness	17.00–18.49	17.00–18.49
Normal range	**18.50–24.99**	**18.50–23.00**
Overweight	**≥25.00**	**>23.00–27.5**
Pre-obese	25.00–29.99	
Obese	**≥30.00**	**>27.5**
Obese class I	30.00–34.99	
Obese class II	35.00–39.99	
Obese class III	≥40.00	

Source: Adapted from Organization WH [56, 64].

Table 4. International classification of adult body mass index.

also be determined by using printed body mass index tables (Appendix C) to using one of the many free smartphone apps.

2.3. Recommendations in special populations

The 1990 IOM recommendations included considerations for "special populations." For instance, women of shorter stature were advised to gain at the lower end of the range for their prepregnant BMI based on their greater risk for emergent cesarean delivery. However, subsequent analyses did not report that this risk was modified by lower PWG.

Other special populations mentioned in the 1990 guidelines were pregnant adolescents, various racial or ethnic groups, and pregnancies with multiple fetuses. The 2009 IOM guidelines obviated the concern of recommending too high PWG in the developmentally normal, slim adolescent by use of the WHO BMI cut-offs in which such adolescents are now classified as normal weight rather than underweight. The 2009 guidelines have provisional guidelines for women with multiple (twins, triplets, etc.) gestations but were not able to address the extremes of prepregnancy BMI such as very high (super obese) or very low prepregnancy BMI categories.

2.3.1. *Twin pregnancy*

Recommended PWG in twin pregnancies is higher than in singleton (single fetus), pregnancies and consistent with singleton pregnancy, is inversely related to prepregnancy BMI category. In other words, a normal-weight woman expecting twins should be advised to gain more than her overweight counterpart expecting twins, but her recommendation is greater than if she was only expecting one baby The IOM was unable to conduct the same level of analysis for women with twins as it did for women with singletons (single fetuses), so the following provisional guidelines were proffered: normal-weight women should gain 17–25 kg (37–54 lbs), overweight women, 14–23 kg (31–50 lbs), and obese women, 11–19 kg (25–42 lbs) during the term [1]. There was insufficient information with which one can develop even a provisional guideline for underweight women with multiple fetuses.

2.3.2. *Prepregnancy extreme obesity*

Obesity at the onset of pregnancy is associated with the increased risk of pregnancy complications (gestational diabetes, hypertension, cesarean delivery) and poorer neonatal outcomes (stillbirth, congenital anomalies) [66, 67]. Since 2006, the increase in adult obesity in developed countries has slowed, but more women in developing countries are obese at the onset of pregnancy [68, 69]. The estimated prevalence of obesity exceeded 50% in women in Kuwait, Kiribati, Federated States of Micronesia, Libya, Qatar, Tonga, and Samoa [70]. Further, there are more women worldwide who are in a BMI category of extreme obesity (≥40 kg/m^2).

Although the 2009 IOM guideline improved upon the 1990 ones in that there was a specific recommendation for obese women (5–9 kg), it was not stratified by the severity of obesity (**Table 3**). This is problematic in that pregnancy and newborn complications increase further in higher categories of obesity [71, 72]. Retrospective studies of pregnant women with severe obesity have been conducted to assess the relationship between degrees of PWG with perinatal outcomes [71–73]. A review of 10 such studies included nearly 740,000 obese women from three countries (United States, Sweden, and Germany). For the outcomes of small for gestational age, large for gestational age, and cesarean delivery, the authors concluded that that PWG guidelines may need modification for the severity of obesity as the lowest combined risk was with weight gain of 5–9 kg in women with class I obesity, from 1 to less than 5 kg for class II obesity, and no gestational weight gain for women with class III obesity [74]. Another review and meta-analysis of 18 studies reported that women in higher obese categories who gained less than the IOM guidelines were less likely to have gestational hypertension, preeclampsia, cesarean delivery, and fewer large for gestational age infants than obese women who gained within the guidelines [75]. In summary, it appears that women in more severely obese categories can safely gain less than the IOM guidelines or even gain minimally overall.

For obese women, it is not uncommon to see weight loss in the first trimester and even up to mid-pregnancy. Besides nausea (with or without vomiting) which may blunt appetite and decrease weight, the "teachable moment" of pregnancy spurs many women to choose food more carefully as they shift their attention to nutritional needs of their growing baby. Weight loss during pregnancy can be alarming to the mother and her family, but the midwife or health worker can provide reassurance that as long as she is well hydrated, some weight loss will not harm her baby. In fact, some obese women improve their nutritional habits enough that they gain well within the guidelines and then after the birth of the infant find themselves to weigh slightly less than they were at the beginning of the pregnancy!

2.3.3. Prepregnancy underweight

Maternal underweight (low BMI) at the onset and during pregnancy is a key determinant of poor fetal outcomes. The prevalence of low BMI is higher in developing nations with suboptimal access to food and greater risk for diarrheal diseases but is also present in developed nations in women with eating disorders or dependence on alcohol or other substances. One such negative outcome is intrauterine growth restriction (IUGR) or low birth weight (LBW, less than 2500 g). IUGR and LBW occur as a result of maternal, placental, and fetal factors [76].

Intrauterine growth restriction is associated with increased perinatal morbidity and mortality, and newborns with low birth weight have increased risk for the development of adult metabolic syndrome. One of the most cited examples of the long-term outcomes of maternal undernutrition is the Dutch Famine Birth Cohort Study [77]. In the winter of 1944/1945 the Nazi occupation turned a once prosperous country to one plagued by famine. Official food rations were below 1000 calories/day resulting in inadequate PWG and low birth weight infants. The offspring have been followed over subsequent decades. As middle-aged adults they were more likely to be obese [78] and have atherogenic lipid profiles [79]. This is explained using the fetal origin hypothesis [27], also referred to as the "thrifty phenotype" hypothesis, in which fetal reprogramming necessary to survive low food availability ended up being a longer-term disadvantage when food was more abundant.

Resting metabolic rate varies among pregnant women. Overweight women enter pregnancy with ample fat stores and their resting metabolism increases in an attempt to diminish further accumulation of fat stores [80]. Conversely, underweight women with limited food supply and the demands of hard physical labor frequently enter pregnancy with minimal maternal fat reserves. Their only option is to reduce their resting metabolic rate to conserve energy for their fetus [81, 82]. This permits delivery of a viable infant who may or may not be growth restricted, depending on the severity of the situation. Such strategies enable women to sustain a pregnancy under a wide range of conditions, including suboptimal nutrition. However, at some point, the physiological capacity of the body to adjust its metabolism and accommodate fetal growth will be compromised; nutrients are preferentially diverted to the mother at the expense of fetal growth.

Health workers may want to consider the positive deviance approach based on the premise that solutions to a community's problem may exist within the community [83]. Positive deviance refers to the uncommon yet healthy practices that permit some persons to thrive while similarly positioned neighbors do not. One example was when program planners in Vietnam observed that mothers who fed their children less typical foods like shrimp and greens from the rice paddies instead of rice only were able to protect them from malnutrition [84]. A similar approach could be taken in communities in which access to sufficient energy, nutrient, and protein stores during pregnancy is suboptimal. There may prove to be "positive deviants" or women who have identified less common but effective means of optimizing pregnancy weight.

http://dx.doi.org/10.5772/intechopen.79066

3. Influences on pregnancy weight gain

Midwives and health workers must consider that there are factors that influence PWG that are modifiable and those which are not modifiable. Further, modifiable factors such as food intake and physical activity are intertwined and are influenced by body habitus and age. It is also critical to be aware that appropriate PWG decreases the risk of pregnancy-related diseases such as gestational hypertension and gestational diabetes.

3.1. Prepregnancy body mass index

Achieving a normal prepregnancy BMI has a significant influence on appropriate PWG [1]. High (obese and overweight) prepregnancy BMI is a recurring key determinant of excessive gain among White [85–88], Black [89], Hispanic [90–93], and multiethnic women [2, 3, 94]. Specifically, overweight BMI has been the most commonly reported determinant of excessive PWG in all ethnicities [2, 4, 31, 88].

As noted previously, more women in developing countries are overweight or obese at the onset of pregnancy [68, 69] and therefore are more likely to have excessive PWG. Globally, the impact of excessive PWG may pose an even greater threat to maternal and infant long-term health in resource-poor settings undergoing various phases of the nutrition transition [95]. The nutrition transition is marked by shifts in diet from traditional foods to a more Western-type diet along with decreasing physical activity that propagates obesity and nutrition-related non-communicable diseases, such as cardiovascular disease and diabetes. As reproductive-age women in these settings were previously exposed to undernutrition and are now becoming overweight/obese, excessive PWG may further lead toward the heightened risk of maternal and offspring obesity and nutrition-related diseases [69].

Conversely, underweight BMI has been implicated in the increased risk of inadequate gain [31] but with less frequency in developed countries. Even with the "globesity epidemic," there are countries like India in which 42% of mothers are underweight and give birth to 20% of the world's babies. In poor-resource areas, women begin pregnancy with low BMI and gain little weight during pregnancy [7].

3.2. Maternal age

Adolescents and younger women [4, 31, 91, 96] are more likely to gain excessively. Though related to concurrent maturation, it is of concern because of the risk of postpartum weight retention and the potential for young women to move to a high BMI category by the next pregnancy [97]. There is less consistency in older women. Deputy et al. [31] reported that inadequate PWG was more likely in multi-ethnic women 35 and older while Puerto Rican women over 30 years of age were at 2.5 times greater risk for excessive PWG than younger women [90].

3.3. Parity

Even one pregnancy changes the fatness of a woman's body. One arm of the CARDIA study showed that White and Black women with a single pregnancy had pregnancy-related increased adiposity as compared to women who remained nulliparous [98]. Parity has a significant relationship to PWG independent of other known influences. In women from England, parity contributed most greatly to PWG followed by birth weight and BMI [85]. Adolescent primiparas gained 5.28 pounds more than multiparas [99]; had twice the likelihood of excessive PWG than multiparas [96]; and large multiethnic studies have also reported primiparity versus subsequent births as a covariate for excessive PWG [2, 3, 100].

3.4. Hypertension and gestational diabetes

A relationship between hypertension in pregnancy and excessive PWG has been observed in women of diverse ethnicities [3, 99, 101, 102]. Midwives and health workers must be aware of both modifiable and non-modifiable factors associated with pregnancy-related hypertension. Compared to White women, Black women consistently have more pregnancy-related hypertension independent of other factors [103–105]. In Hispanics, findings are less consistent: from reports of lower risk [106] to differential risk, higher risk for certain types of hypertension (e.g., preeclampsia but not gestational hypertension) [107]. In all ethnicities, pregnancy-related hypertension is more common in primiparas [102] and in women with a family history of hypertension [108].

High prepregnancy BMI and excessive PWG are modifiable factors that appear to have independent as well as synergistic influences on hypertension in pregnancy. Women with excessive PWG had a three-fold risk of hypertension and four-fold risk of preeclampsia compared to women who gained appropriately [109], and women with obese BMI had 2.5-fold higher odds of having pregnancy-related hypertension with excessive PWG compared to those who gained adequately [110].

Increased risk for gestational diabetes mellitus is associated with excessive PWG in early pregnancy [111]. However, once diagnosed with gestational diabetes, women may be more likely to gain inadequately [92, 93] or adequately [90] overall due to dietary and exercise modifications. Therefore, the diagnosis of gestational diabetes is really an opportunity to optimize pregnancy health through monitoring dietary intake and being more intentional to add physical activity as a means of controlling blood-sugar levels.

4. Postpartum effects of excessive pregnancy weight gain

Excessive PWG in women of all prepregnancy BMI categories exerts negative effects on the mother and her infant. Women with excessive gain are at greater risk for cesarean delivery [14–16] and more likely to have pregnancy complications [15]. Infants of women with excessive PWG are more likely to be overweight by 7 years of age [22] and to be obese by adolescence [25]. If this adolescent is female, then she begins pregnancy in a high BMI and is already at greater risk for excessive PWG. After delivery, women with excessive PWG are more prone to postpartum weight retention [11, 17] and more likely to become overweight or obese by the next pregnancy [19, 112, 113].

Postpartum weight retention is defined as the weight change from preconception to the first year postpartum. Postpartum weight retention includes PWG, the early postpartum weight loss (from delivery to 6 weeks of postpartum), and late postpartum loss (subsequent weight changes in the postpartum year [114]. Early postpartum weight loss is from the combined weight of the infant, placenta, amniotic fluid, and water accumulated during pregnancy. Depending on the size of the infant and amount of water accumulated, the loss will be about 7 kg (15 lb). However, with an average PWG of 12–14 kg, 4–6 kg is the maternal fat gain, often referred to as "baby fat." Therefore, late postpartum weight loss requires loss of maternal fat that was acquired to support the pregnancy. With excessive PWG, there is even greater fat deposition and the mother has yet more weight to lose.

The pattern of postpartum weight changes was examined in multi-ethnic women (n = 985) aged 18–41 years with 2 consecutive births between 1980 and 1990 [18]. Early postpartum weight change (6 weeks of postpartum) was similar in all four groups. However, the underweight and normal-weight groups lost more late postpartum weight even though their average PWG was greater. The higher (overweight and obese) BMI groups gained less during pregnancy but had diminished weight loss in the later postpartum period. This demonstrated that early postpartum loss is simply a reversal of physiological processes of pregnancy but late postpartum loss requires an alteration in maternal fat stores.

Another multi-ethnic study of young women aged 14–25 years (n = 427) reported that nearly two-thirds had excessive PWG. Of those, 33% of the young women moved to a higher BMI category in the first-year postpartum resulting in 68% being overweight or obese [97].

Excessive PWG is the single greatest contributor to postpartum weight retention and subsequent life-long obesity and related co-morbidities [19, 113]. However, this is further compounded by acculturation/globalization, for example, acquisition of Western patterns of eating and more sedentary work [68, 69, 115]; ethnicity, as women of color are less likely to lose postpartum weight or to gain weight in the postpartum period [116, 117]; short interpregnancy interval [118]; and lower socioeconomic status [119].

Obviously, diminishing postpartum weight retention is greatly dependent on gaining appropriately during pregnancy and not "eating for two." Health workers and midwives should prepare pregnant women for exclusive breastfeeding for at least 6 months not only for the well-known health benefits to the baby but for the increased metabolic expenditure needed for lactation [120]. In women who exclusively breastfed for even 6 months, postpartum weight retention was eliminated in women with average PWG and any weight gain was reduced in all but women with BMI ≥35 kg/m^2 [121]. Each additional week of breastfeeding resulted in an additional postpartum loss or 1.5 lb [97]. In the longer term, breastfeeding has effects on the mother's health beyond postpartum. Middle-aged women who never breastfed were compared to those who breastfed for even 3 months and had waist circumferences of 6.5 cm greater, 28% more central obesity, and therefore greater risk for cardiovascular disease [122].

Therefore, beyond the direct positive effect on postpartum weight retention, and the benefits to the infant, breastfeeding positively influences the mother's trajectory of cardiovascular risk.

5. Conclusions

Achieving appropriate pregnancy weight gain is necessary to optimize maternal, infant, and population health but it is not easily done. Promoting healthy weight gain during pregnancy is an investment in both the mother's longevity and the next generation. As health workers, we see the individual and societal outcomes when women gain too much or too little in pregnancy. Women who gain too much suffer the health consequences from obesity and its associated morbidities. Women who gain suboptimally have infants with more susceptibility to disease and death. The platform of excessive pregnancy weight gain is that up to 50% of women in certain countries start pregnancy overweight or obese. Though the first wave of obesity seen in developed countries is slowing, the developing countries have now taken the globesity baton as they transition to Western eating and more sedentary lifestyles. Women who are young, in their first pregnancy, and who start pregnancy with a high body mass index are much more likely to gain excessively and their more complicated pregnancies come at a cost to their health in the short term and long term. Women who do not have proper access to food and start pregnancy undernourished may ultimately not be able to supply the necessary nutrients for optimal growth and development of their infant.

During pregnancy, it is customary for women to solicit and process advice. Pregnancy weight gain is a topic in which women must receive advice that is based on evidence. As health workers we are the source of this evidence, whether from a local ministry of health or from a weight gain guideline that is recognized as applicable to women of your area. Basic pregnancy weight gain guidelines are as follows: women who are underweight or normal weight need to gain more pregnancy weight than do overweight and obese women. Overweight and obese women do not need additional fat stores as do women in lower BMI categories. Most of the weight gained in pregnancy should be from mid-pregnancy to term as this is the period of fetal growth. In early pregnancy, some women may not gain any weight or may even lose some weight. This is acceptable as long as there are no signs of dehydration or disease. All women need a balance of energy and protein in the second and third trimesters for the rapidly developing fetus. Avoiding excessive gain will dramatically lessen the chance of retaining weight during postpartum and ending up in a high BMI category by the next pregnancy. Exclusive breastfeeding for at least 6 months benefits the infant, increases maternal metabolism and has protective effects for cardiovascular disease in middle age. Pregnancy weight gain is important in the short term and in the long term.

Conflict of interest

I have no financial interests to disclose.

Notes/thanks/other declarations

I must recognize the army of doctors, midwives and health workers who strive to make birth safer for the women and babies of the world. Thank you for doing much with little and for your joy in this wonderful work that we are blessed to do!

A. Appendix

Nutritional Interventions for a Positive Pregnancy		
Dietary interventions	Counselling about healthy eating and keeping physically active during pregnancy is recommended for pregnant women to stay healthy and to prevent excessive weight gain during pregnancy. Note: A healthy diet contains adequate energy, protein, vitamins and minerals, obtained through the consumption of a variety of foods, including green and orange vegetables, meat, fish, beans, nuts, whole grains and fruit.	Recommended
	In undernourished populations, nutrition education on increasing daily energy and protein intake is recommended for pregnant women to reduce the risk of low-birth-weight neonates.	Context-specific recommendation
	In undernourished populations, balanced energy and protein dietary supplementation is recommended for pregnant women to reduce the risk of stillbirths and small-for-gestational-age neonates.	Context-specific recommendation
	In undernourished populations, high-protein supplementation is not recommended for pregnant women to improve maternal and perinatal outcomes.	Not recommended
Iron and folic acid supplements	Daily oral iron and folic acid supplementation with 30 mg to 60 mg of elemental iron and 400 g (0.4 mg) of folic acid is recommended for pregnant women to prevent maternal anemia, puerperal sepsis, low birth weight, and preterm birth.	Recommended
	Intermittent oral iron and folic acid supplementation with 120 mg of elemental iron and 2800 g (2.8 mg) of folic acid once weekly is recommended for pregnant women to improve maternal and neonatal outcomes if daily iron is not acceptable due to side-effects, and in populations with an anemia prevalence among pregnant women of less than 20%.	Context-specific recommendation
Calcium supplements	In populations with low dietary calcium intake, daily calcium supplementation (1.5–2.0 g oral elemental calcium) is recommended for pregnant women to reduce the risk of pre-eclampsia.	Context-specific recommendation
Vitamin A supplements	Vitamin A supplementation is only recommended for pregnant women in areas where vitamin A deficiency is a severe public health problem to prevent night blindness.	Context-specific Recommendation

Adapted from: World Health Organization. WHO recommendations on antenatal care for a positive pregnancy experience. Geneva, Switzerland: WHO Press; 2016. p. 14 *Summary list of WHO recommendations on antenatal care (ANC) for a positive pregnancy* experience.

B. Appendix

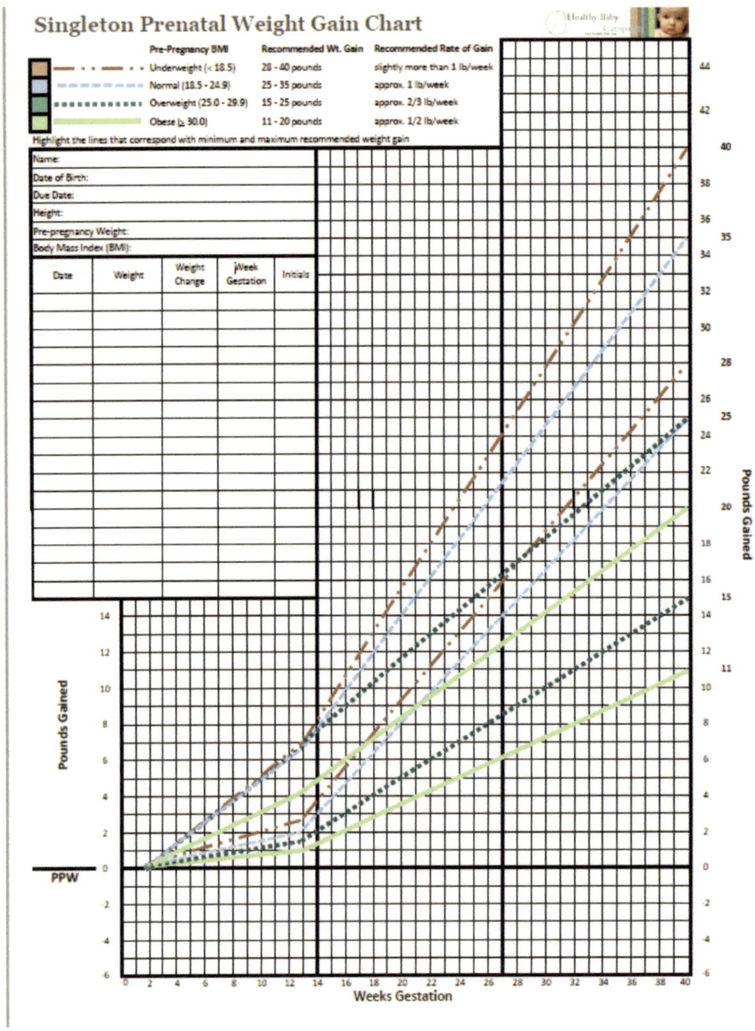

Colorado Department of Health Care Policy and Financing. Prenatal Plus Program 2018 [Available from: https://www.colorado.gov/pacific/hcpf/prenatal-plus-program].

Colorado Department of Health Care Policy and Financing [54].

http://dx.doi.org/10.5772/intechopen.79066

C. Appendix

BMI Chart:

American Institute for Cancer Research; "Heal Well Guide 2013"

Height	Weight	Weight in Pounds (without clothes)												
4'11"	*94<*	*99*	*104*	*109*	*114*	*119*	*124*	*128*	*133*	*138*	*143*	*148*	*173*	*198*
5'	97	102	107	112	118	123	128	133	138	143	148	153	179	204
5'1"	100	106	111	116	122	127	132	137	143	148	153	158	185	211
5'2"	104	109	115	120	126	131	136	142	147	153	158	164	191	218
5'3"	107	113	118	124	130	135	141	146	152	158	163	169	197	225
5'4"	110	116	122	128	134	140	145	151	157	163	169	174	204	232
5'5"	114	120	126	132	138	144	150	156	162	168	174	180	210	240
5'6"	118	124	130	136	142	148	155	161	167	173	179	186	216	247
5'7"	121	127	134	140	146	153	159	166	172	178	185	191	223	255
5'8"	125	131	138	144	151	158	164	171	177	184	190	197	230	262
5'9"	128	135	142	149	155	162	169	176	182	189	196	203	236	270
5'10"	132	139	146	153	160	167	174	181	188	195	202	207	243	278
5'11"	136	143	150	157	165	172	179	186	193	200	208	215	250	286
6'	140	147	154	162	169	177	184	191	199	206	213	221	258	294
6'1"	144	151	159	166	174	182	189	197	204	212	219	227	265	302
6'2"	148	155	163	171	179	186	194	202	210	218	225	233	272	311
BMI	19	20	21	22	23	24	25	26	27	28	29	30	35	40

Author details

Ruth Mielke

Address all correspondence to: ruthmielke@fullerton.edu

California State University, Fullerton, Fullerton, California, United States

References

[1] Institute of Medicine. Weight Gain during Pregnancy: Reexamining the Guidelines. Washington, D.C.: National Academy Press; 2009

[2] Brawarsky P, Stotland NE, Jackson RA, Fuentes-Afflick E, Escobar G, Rubashkin N, et al. Pre-pregnancy and pregnancy-related factors and the risk of excessive or inadequate gestational weight gain. International Journal of Gynecology & Obstetrics. 2005;**91**:125-131

[3] Wells CS, Schwalberg R, Noonan G, Gabor V. Factors influencing inadequate and excessive weight gain in pregnancy: Colorado, 2000-2002. Maternal and Child Health Journal. 2006;**10**(1):55-62

[4] Schieve LA, Cogswell ME, Scanlon KS. Trends in pregnancy weight gain within and outside ranges recommended by the Institute of Medicine in a WIC population. Maternal and Child Health Journal. 1998;**2**(2):111-116

[5] Gao X, Yan Y, Xiang S, Zeng G, Liu S, Sha T, et al. The mutual effect of pre-pregnancy body mass index, waist circumference and gestational weight gain on obesity-related adverse pregnancy outcomes: A birth cohort study. PLoS One. 2017;**12**(6):1-13

[6] Sae Kyung C, Guisera L, Yeon Hee K, In Yang P, Hyun Sun K, Jong Chul S. Determining optimal gestational weight gain in the Korean population: A retrospective cohort study. Reproductive Biology and Endocrinology. 2017;**15**:1-7

[7] Coffey D. Prepregnancy body mass and weight gain during pregnancy in India and sub-Saharan Africa. Proceedings of the National Academy of Sciences. 2015;**112**(11):3302-3307

[8] Young MF, Hong Nguyen P, Addo OY, Pham H, Nguyen S, Martorell R, et al. Timing of gestational weight gain on fetal growth and infant size at birth in Vietnam. PLoS One. 2017;**12**(1):1-11

[9] Acharya O, Zotor FB, Chaudhary P, Deepak K, Amuna P, Ellahi B. Maternal nutritional status, food intake and pregnancy weight gain in Nepal. Journal of Health Management. 2016;**18**(1):1-12

[10] Han Z, Lutsiv O, Mulla S, Rosen A, Beyene J, McDonald SD. Low gestational weight gain and the risk of preterm birth and low birthweight: A systematic review and meta-analyses. Acta Obstetricia et Gynecologica Scandinavica. 2011;**90**(9):935-954

[11] Siega-Riz AM, Viswanathan M, Moos M-K, Deierlein A, Mumford S, Knaack J, et al. A systematic review of outcomes of maternal weight gain according to the Institute of Medicine recommendations: Birthweight, fetal growth, and postpartum weight retention. American Journal of Obstetrics and Gynecology. 2009;**201**(4):339.e1-339e14

[12] Chung JGY, Taylor RS, Thompson JMD, Anderson NH, Dekker GA, Kenny LC, et al. Gestational weight gain and adverse pregnancy outcomes in a nulliparous cohort. European Journal of Obstetrics and Gynecology and Reproductive Biology. 2013;**167**(2):149-153

[13] Davis RR, Hofferth SL, Shenassa ED. Gestational weight gain and risk of infant death in the United States. American Journal of Public Health. 2014;**104**(S1):S90-SS5

[14] Stotland NE, Hopkins LM, Caughey AB. Gestational weight gain, macrosomia, and the risk of cesarean birth in nondiabetic nulliparas. Obstetrics and Gynecology. 2004;**104**:671-677

[15] DeVader SR, Neeley HL, Myles TD, Leet TL. Evaluation of gestation weight gain guidelines for women with normal prepregnancy body mass index. Obstetrics and Gynecology. 2007;**110**(4):745-751

[16] Rhodes JC, Schoendorf KC, Parker JD. Contribution of excess weight during pregnancy and macrosomia to the cesarean delivery rate. Pediatrics. 2003;**111**(5):1181-1185

[17] Gore SA, Brown DM, West DS. The role of postpartum weight retention in obesity among women: A review of the evidence. Annals of Behavioral Medicine: A Publication of the Society of Behavioral Medicine. 2003;**26**(2):149-159

[18] Gunderson EP, Abrams B, Selvin S. Does the pattern of postpartum weight change differ according to pregravid body size? International Journal of Obesity and Related Metabolic Disorders: Journal of the International Association for the Study of Obesity. 2001;**25**(6):853-862

[19] Rooney BL, Schauberger CW. Excess pregnancy weight gain and long-term obesity: One decade later. Obstetrics and Gynecology. 2002;**100**(2):245-252

[20] Schmitt N, Nicholson W, Schmitt J. The association of pregnancy and the development of obesity—Results of a systematic review and meta-analysis on the natural history of post-partum weight retention. International Journal of Obesity (London). 2007;**31**:1642-1651

[21] Salsberry PJ, Reagan PB. The dynamics of early childhood overweight. Pediatrics. 2005;**116**(6):1329-1338

[22] Wrotniak BH, Shults J, Butts S, Stettler N. Gestational weight gain and risk of overweight in the offspring at age 7 y in a multicenter, multiethnic cohort study. The American Journal of Clinical Nutrition. 2008;**87**(6):1818-1824

[23] Oken E, Taveras EM, Kleinman KP, Rich-Edwards JW, Gillman MW. Gestational weight gain and child adiposity at age 3 years. American Journal of Obstetrics and Gynecology. 2007;**196**(4):322.e1-322.e8

[24] Salsberry PJ, Reagan PB. Taking the long view: The prenatal environment and early adolescent overweight. Research in Nursing and Health. 2007;**30**:297-307

[25] Oken E, Rifas-Shiman SL, Field AE, Frazier AL, Gillman MW. Maternal gestational weight gain and offspring weight in adolescence. Obstetrics and Gynecology. 2008;**112**(5):999-1006. DOI: 10.97/AOG.0b013e31818a5d50

[26] Lau C, Rogers JM, Desai M, Ross MG. Fetal programming of adult disease: Implications for prenatal care. Obstetrics and Gynecology. 2011;**117**(4):978-985

[27] Barker DJP. The developmental origins of adult disease. Journal of the American College of Nutrition. 2004;**23**(suppl_6):588S-5895S

[28] Hytten FE. Weight gain in pregnancy. In: Hytten FE, Chamberlain G, editors. Clinical Physiology in Obstetrics. London: Blackwell Scientific Publications; 1991

[29] King JC. Physiology of pregnancy and nutrient metabolism. The American Journal of Clinical Nutrition. 2000;**71**(5):1218S-1225S

[30] World Health Organization. WHO Recommendations on Antenatal Care for a Positive Pregnancy Experience. Geneva, Switzerland: WHO Press; 2016

[31] Deputy NPMPH, Sharma AJPMPH, Kim SYMPH, Hinkle SNP. Prevalence and characteristics associated with gestational weight gain adequacy. Obstetrics and Gynecology. 2015;**125**(4):773-781

[32] KTL, Aikins MP. Evidence-based approaches to managing nausea and vomiting in early pregnancy. Journal of Midwifery and Women's Health. 2009;**54**(6):430-444

[33] Cunningham F, Leveno K, Bloom S, Hauth J, Spong C, Dashe J. Williams Obstetrics. 24th ed. New York: McGraw-Hill Professional Publishing; 2014

[34] Lain KY, Catalano PM. Metabolic changes in pregnancy. Clinical Obstetrics and Gynecology. 2007;**50**(4):938-948. DOI: 10.1097/GRF.0b013e31815a5494

[35] King TL, Davidson MR, Avery MD, Anderson CM. Anatomy and physiology of pregnancy: Placental, fetal, and maternal adaptations. In: King T, Brucker M, Kriebs J, Fahey J, Gegor C, Varney H, editors. Varney's Midwifery. 5th ed. Burlington, MA: Jones & Bartlett Learning; 2015. pp. 599-627

[36] Botehlo N, Emeis CL, Brucker MC. Gastrointestinal conditions. In: Brucker MC, King TL, editors. Pharmacology for Women's Health. 2nd ed. Burlington, MA: Jones & Bartlett; 2017. p. 605-642

[37] Lewallen LP. Healthy behaviors and sources of health information among low-income pregnant women. Public Health Nursing. 2004;**21**(3):200-206

[38] McBride CM, Emmons KM, Lipkus IM. Understanding the potential of teachable moments: The case of smoking cessatoin. Health Education Research. 2003;**18**(2):156-170

[39] Phelan S. Pregnancy: A "teachable moment" for weight control and obesity prevention. American Journal of Obstetrics and Gynecology. 2010;**202**(2):135.e1-135.e8

[40] Liu J, Whitaker KM, Yu SM, Chao SM, Lu MC. Association of provider advice and pregnancy weight gain in a predominantly Hispanic population. Women's Health Issues. 2016;**26**(3):321-328

[41] Chesley LC. Hypertension in pregnancy: Definitions, familial factor, and remote prognosis. Kidney International. 1980;**18**(2):234-240

[42] ACOG. Hypertension in pregnancy: Executive summary. Obstetrics and Gynecology. 2013;**122**(5):1122-1131

[43] Ota E, Hori H, Mori R, Tobe-Gai R, Farrar D. Antenatal dietary education and supplementation to increase energy and protein intake. Cochrane Database of Systematic Reviews. 2015;(6):CD000032

[44] Ghosh S, Suri D, Uauy R. Assessment of protein adequacy in developing countries: Quality matters. British Journal of Nutrition. 2012;**108**(S2):S77-S87

[45] Kinoshita T. Longitudinal variance of fat mass deposition during pregnancy evaluated by ultrasonography: The ratio of visceral fat to subcutaneous fat in the abdomen. Gynecologic and Obstetric Investigation. 2006;**61**(2):115-118

[46] Wyness L, Stanner S, Buttriss J, British Nutrition Foundation S. Nutrition and Development : Short and Long Term Consequences for Health. Chicester, United Kingdom: John Wiley & Sons, Incorporated; 2013

[47] Jansson T, Powell TL. Human placental transport in altered fetal growth: Does the placenta function as a nutrient sensor?- A Review. Placenta. 2006;**27**:91-97

[48] Institute of Medicine. Nutrition in Pregnancy: Part 1-Weight Gain. Medicine Io, editor. Washington, D.C.: National Academy Press; 1990. 1-233 pp

[49] Fernandez ID, Olson CM, De Ver Dye T. Discordance in the assessment of prepregnancy weight status of adolescents: A comparison between the Centers for Disease Control and Prevention sex- and age-specific body mass index classification and the Institute of Medicine-based classification used for maternal weight gain guidelines. Journal of the American Dietetic Association. 2008;**108**(6):998-1002

[50] Groth S. Are the Institute of Medicine recommendations for gestational weight gain appropriate for adolescents. Journal of Obstetric, Gynecologic, and Neonatal Nursing: JOGNN/NAACOG. 2007;**36**(1):21-27

[51] Picciano MF. Pregnancyand lactation: Physiological adjustments, nutrtitional requirements and the role of dietary supplements. The Journal of Nutrition. 2003;**133**(Suppl): 1997-2002

[52] Organization WH. Good maternal nutrition: The best start in life Copenhagen, Denmark: WHO Regional Office for Europe; 2016. Available from: http://www.euro.who.int/__data/assets/pdf_file/0008/313667/Good-maternal-nutrition-The-best-start-in-life.pdf?ua=1

[53] Francisco M, Pedro R. A weight gain chart for pregnant women designed in Chile. Maternal and Child Nutrition. 2005;**1**(2):77-90

[54] Godoy AC, do Nascimento SL, Surita FG. A systematic review and meta-analysis of gestational weight gain recommendations and related outcomes in Brazil. Clinics. 2015;**70**(11):758-764

[55] Colorado Department of Health Care Policy and Financing. Prenatal Plus Program 2018. Available from: https://www.colorado.gov/pacific/hcpf/prenatal-plus-program

[56] Prenatal Weight Gain Grids [Forms]. Los Angeles: Los Angeles County Department of Public Health; 1990. Available from: http://www.lapublichealth.org/mch/cpsp/cpsp-forms.htm

[57] WHO Expert Consultation. Appropriate body-mass index for Asian populations and its implications for policy and intervention strategies. The Lancet. 2004;**363**(9403):157-163

[58] Xin ET, Carson AJ, Rahul M, Huishan K, Truls Ø, Chye TT. Determining optimal gestational weight gain in a multiethnic Asian population. Journal of Obstetrics and Gynaecology Research. 2014;**40**(4):1002-1008

[59] Ota E, Haruna M, Suzuki M, Anh DD, Tho LH, Tam NTT, et al. Maternal body mass index and gestational weight gain and their association with perinatal outcomes in Viet Nam. Bulletin of the World Health Organization. 2011;**89**(2):127-136

[60] Jih J, Mukherjea A, Vittinghoff E, Nguyen TT, Tsoh JY, Fukuoka Y, et al. Using appropriate body mass index cut points for overweight and obesity among Asian Americans. Preventive Medicine. 2014;**65**:1-6

[61] Nomura K, Kido M, Tanabe A, Nagashima K, Takenoshita S, Ando K. Investigation of optimal weight gain during pregnancy for Japanese women. Scientific Reports. 2017;**7**:2569

[62] Jill C, Michael C, Diana G, Polly B. Who should be estimating a patient's weight in the emergency department? Academic Emergency Medicine. 2005;**12**(3):262-266

[63] Nguyen T, Gupta A, Quiros M, Davidson T, Hasandzekaj A, Akhtar S, et al. 225 accuracy of patient weight estimations in the emergency department by emergency department providers. Annals of Emergency Medicine. 2011;**58**(4, Suppl):S252-S2S3

[64] Widen EM, Gallagher D. Body composition changes in pregnancy: Measurement, predictors and outcomes. European Journal of Clinical Nutrition. 2014;**68**(6):643-652

[65] Organization WH. Global database on body mass index: BMI classifications 2011. Available from: http://www.assessmentpsychology.com/icbmi.htm

[66] ACOG. Practice bulletin no 156: Obesity in pregnancy. Obstetrics and Gynecology. 2015;**126**(6):e112-ee26

[67] Lim CC, Mahmood T. Obesity in pregnancy. Best Practice and Research Clinical Obstetrics and Gynaecology. 2015;**29**(3):309-319

[68] Mendez MA, Monteiro CA, Popkin BM. Overweight exceeds underweight among women in most developing countries. The American Journal of Clinical Nutrition. 2005;**81**(3):714-721

[69] Costa-Font J, Mas N. 'Globesity'? The effects of globalization on obesity and caloric intake. Food Policy. 2016;**64**:121-132

[70] Ng M, Fleming T, Robinson M, Thomson B, Graetz N, Margono C, et al. Global, regional, and national prevalence of overweight and obesity in children and adults during 1980-2013: A systematic analysis for the Global Burden of Disease Study 2013. The Lancet. 2014;**9945**:766-781

[71] Bodnar LM, Siega-Riz AM, Simhan HN, Himes KP, Abrams B. Severe obesity, gestational weight gain, and adverse birth outcomes. The American Journal of Clinical Nutrition. 2010;**91**(6):1642-1648

[72] Swank ML, Marshall NE, Caughey AB, Main EK, Gilbert WM, Melsop KA, et al. Pregnancy outcomes in the super obese, stratified by weight gain above and below Institute of Medicine guidelines. Obstetrics and Gynecology. 2014;**124**(6):1105-1110

[73] Kiel DW, Dodson EA, Artal R, Boehmer TK. Gestational weight gain and pregnancy outcomes in obese women. Obstetrics and Gynecology. 2007;**110**(7):752-758

[74] Faucher MA, Barger MK. Gestational weight gain in obese women by class of obesity and select maternal/newborn outcomes: A systematic review. Women and Birth. 2015;**28**(3):e70-ee9

[75] Kapadia MZ, Park CK, Beyene J, Giglia L, Maxwell C, McDonald SD. Can we safely recommend gestational weight gain below the 2009 guidelines in obese women? A systematic review and meta-analysis. Obesity Reviews. 2015;**16**(3):189-206

[76] Brodsky D, Christou H. Current concepts in intrauterine growth restriction. Journal of Intensive Care Medicine. 2004;**19**(6):307-319

[77] Susser M. Prenatal nutrition, birthweight, and psychological development: An overview of experiements, quasi-experiments, and natural experiments in the past decade. The American Journal of Clinical Nutrition. 1981;**34**:784-803

[78] Ravelli ACJ, van der Meulen JHP, Osmond C, Barker DJP, Bleker O. Obesity at the age of 50 y in men and women exposed to famine prenatally. American Journal of Clinical Nutrition. 1999;**70**:811-816

[79] Roseboom TJ, van der Meulen JH, Osmond C, Barker DJ, Ravelli AC, Bleker OP. Plasma lipid profiles in adults after prenatal exposure to the Dutch famine. American Journal of Clinical Nutrition. 2000;**72**(5):1101-1106

[80] Bronstein MN, Mak RP, King JC. Unexpected relationship between fat mass and basal metabolic rate in pregnant women. British Journal of Nutrition. 1996;**75**:659-668

[81] Poppitt SD, Prentice AM, Jéquier E, Schutz Y, Whitehead RG. Evidence of energy sparing in Gambian women during pregnancy: A longitudinal study using whole-body calorimetry. The American Journal of Clinical Nutrition. 1993;**57**(3):353-364

[82] Melzer K, Schutz Y, Soehnchen N, Othenin Girard V, Martinez De Tejada B, Pichard C, et al. Prepregnancy body mass index and resting metabolic rate during pregnancy. Annals of Nutrition and Metabolism. 2011;**57**(3-4):221-227

[83] Marsh DR, Schoeder DG, Dearden KA, Sternin J, Sternin M. The power of positive deviance. British Medical Journal. 2004;**13**:1177-1179

[84] Mackintosh UAT, Marsh DR, Schroeder DG. Sustained positive deviant child care practices and their effects on child growth in Viet Nam. Food and Nutrition Bulletin. 2002;**23**(Suppl 4):16-25

[85] Harris HE, Ellison GT, Holliday M. Is there an independent association between parity and maternal weight gain? Annals of Human Biology. 1997;**24**(6):507-519

[86] Olson C, Strawderman M. Modifiable behavioral factors in a biopsychosocial model predict inadequate and excessive gestational weight gain. The Journal of the American Dietetic Association. 2003;**103**:48-54

[87] Strychar IM, Chabot C, Champagne F, Ghadirian P, Leduc L, Lemonnier MC, et al. Psychosocial and lifestyle factors associated with insufficient and excessive maternal weight gain during pregnancy. Journal of the American Dietetic Association. 2000;**100**(3):353-356

[88] Olafsdottir AS, Skuladottir GV, Thorsdottir I, Hauksson A, Steingrimsdottir L. Maternal diet in early and late pregnancy in relation to weight gain. International Journal Of Obesity (2005). 2006;**30**(3):492-499

[89] Lederman SA, Alfasi G, Deckelbaum RJ. Pregnancy-associated obesity in black women in New York City. Maternal and Child Health Journal. 2002;**6**(1):37-42

[90] Chasan-Taber L, Schmidt MD, Pekow P, Sternfeld B, Solomon CG, Markenson G. Predictors of excessive and inadequate gestational weight gain in Hispanic women. Obesity (Silver Spring, Md). 2008;**16**(7):1657-1666

[91] Koleilat M, Whaley S. Trends and predictors of excessive gestational weight gain among Hispanic WIC participants in Southern California. Maternal and Child Health Journal. 2013;**17**(8):1399-1404

[92] Walker LO, Hoke MM, Brown A. Risk factors for excessive or inadequate gestational weight gain among Hispanic women in a U.S.-Mexico border state. Journal of Obstetric, Gynecologic, and Neonatal Nursing. 2009;**38**(4):418-429

[93] Mielke R, Gorman N. Predictors of gestational weight gain in Mexican American women in Los Angeles. Californian Journal of Health Promotion. 2015;**13**(3):1-18

[94] Walker LO, Kim M. Psychosocial thriving during late pregnancy: Relationship to ethnicity, gestational weight gain, and birth weight. Journal of Obstetric, Gynecologic and Neonatal Nursing: JOGNN/NAACOG. 2002;**31**(3):263-274

[95] Popkin BM. Technology, transport, globalization and the nutrition transition food policy. Food Policy. 2006;**31**(6):554-569

[96] Howie LD, Parker JD, Schoendorf KC. Excessive maternal weight gain patterns in adolescents. Journal of the American Dietetic Association. 2003;**103**(12):1653-1657

[97] Gould Rothberg EB, Magriples U, Kershaw TS, Rising SS, Ickovics JR. Gestational weight gain and subsequent postpartum weight loss among young, low-income, ethnic minority women. American Journal of Obstetrics and Gynecology. 2011;**204**(1):52.e1-52e11

[98] Smith DE, Lewis CE, Caveny LL, Perkins GL, Burke GL, Bild DE. Longitudinal changes in adiposity associated with pregnancy. The CARDIA study. Coronary Artery Risk Development in Young Adults Study. JAMA. 1994;**271**(22):151-158

[99] Scholl TO, Salmon RW, Miller LK, Vasilenko P, Furey CH, Christine M. Weight gain during adolescent pregnancy. Associated maternal characteristics and effects on birth weight. Journal of Adolescent Health Care: Official Publication of the Society for Adolescent Medicine. 1988;**9**(4):286-290

[100] Abrams B, Parker JD. Maternal weight gain in women with good pregnancy outcome. Obstetrics and Gynecology. 1990;**76**(1):1-7

[101] Caulfield LE, Witter FR, Stoltzfus R. Determinants of gestational weight gain outside the recommended ranges among white and black women. Obstetrics and Gynecology. 1996;**87**(5):760-766

[102] Johnson J, Clifton RG, Roberts JM, Myatt L, Hauth JC, Spong CY, et al. Pregnancy outcomes with weight gain above or below the 2009 Institute of Medicine guidelines. Obstetrics and Gynecology. 2013;**121**(5):969-975

[103] Chappell LC, Enye S, Seed P, Briley AL, Poston L, Shennan A. Adverse perinatal outcomes and risk factors for preeclampsia in women with chronic hypertension—A prospective study. Hypertension. 2008;**51**(4):1002-1009

[104] Knuist M, Bonsel GJ, Zondervan HA, Treffers PE. Risk factors for preeclampsia in nulliparous women in distinct ethnic groups: A prospective cohort study. Obstetrics and Gynecology. 1998;**92**(2):174-178

[105] Liu J, Gallagher AE, Carta CM, Torres ME, Moran R, Wilcox S. Racial differences in gestational weight gain and pregnancy-related hypertension. Annals of Epidemiology. 2014;**24**(6):441-447

[106] Yeo S, Wells P, Kieffer E, Nolan G. Preeclampsia among Hispanic women in a Detroit health system. Ethnicity and Disease. 2007;**17**(1):118-121

[107] Wolf M, Shah A, Jimenez-Kimble R, Sauk J, Ecker JL, Thadhani R. Differential risk of hypertensive disorders of pregnancy among Hispanic women. The Journal of the American Society of Nephrology. 2004;**15**(5):1330-1338

[108] Ness BR, Markovic MN, Bass MD, Harger MG, Roberts MJ. Family history of hypertension, heart disease, and stroke among women who develop hypertension in pregnancy. Obstetrics and Gynecology. 2003;**102**(6):1366-1371

[109] Fortner RT, Pekow P, Solomon CG, Markenson G, Chasan-Taber L. Prepregnancy body mass index, gestational weight gain, and risk of hypertensive pregnancy among Latina women. American Journal of Obstetrics and Gynecology. 2009;**200**(2):167.e1-167.e7

[110] Chandrasekaran S, Levine LD, Durnwald CP, Elovitz MA, Srinivas SK. Excessive weight gain and hypertensive disorders of pregnancy in the obese patient. The Journal of Maternal-Fetal & Neonatal Medicine. 2015;**28**(8):964-968

[111] Carreno CA, Clifton RG, Hauth JC, Myatt L, Roberts JM, Spong CY, et al. Excessive early gestational weight gain and risk of gestational diabetes mellitus in nulliparous women. Obstetrics and Gynecology. 2012;**119**(6):1227-1233

[112] Gunderson EP, Abrams B, Selvin S. The relative importance of gestational gain and maternal characteristics associated with the risk of becoming overweight after pregnancy. International Journal of Obesity. 2000;**24**:1660-1668

[113] Rooney BL, Schauberger CW, Mathiason MA. Impact of perinatal weight change on long-term obesity and obesity related illnesses. Obstetrics and Gynecology. 2005;**106**(6):1349-1356

[114] Gunderson EP. Childbearing and obesity in women: Weight before, during, and after pregnancy. Obstetrics and Gynecology Clinics of North America. 2009;**36**(2):317-332

[115] Gutierrez YM. Cultural factors affecting diet and pregnancy outcome of pregnant adolescents. Journal of Adolescent Health. 1999;**25**:227-237

[116] Boardley DJ, Sargent RG, Coker AL, Hussey JR, Sharpe PA. The relationship between diet, activity, and other factors, and postpartum weight change by race. Obstetrics and Gynecology. 1995;**86**(5):834-838

[117] Walker L, Freeland-Graves JH, Milani T, George G, Hanss-Nuss H, Kim M, et al. Weight and behavioral and psychosocial factors among ethinically diverse, low-income women after childbirth: II. Trends and correlates. Women and Health. 2004;**40**(2):19-34

[118] Davis E, Babineau D, Wang X, Zyzanski S, Abrams B, Bodnar L, et al. Short inter-pregnancy intervals, parity, excessive pregnancy weight gain and risk of maternal obesity. Maternal and Child Health Journal. 2014;**18**(3):554-562

[119] Shrewsbury V, Robb K, Power C, Wardle J. Socioeconomic differences in weight retention, weight-related attitudes and practices in postpartum women. Maternal and Child Health Journal. 2009;**13**(2):231-240

[120] Butte NF, Hopkinson JM, Mehta N, Moon JK, Smith EOB. Adjustments in energy expenditure and substrate utilization during late pregnancy and lactation. The American Journal of Clinical Nutrition. 1999;**69**(2):299-307

[121] Baker JL, Gamborg M, Heitmann BL, Lissner L, Sørensen TI, Rasmussen KM. Breastfeeding reduces postpartum weight retention. The American Journal of Clinical Nutrition. 2008;**88**(6):1543-1551

[122] McClure CK, Schwarz EB, Conroy MB, Tepper PG, Janssen I, Sutton-Tyrrell KC. Breastfeeding and subsequent maternal visceral adiposity. Obesity. 2011;**19**(11): 2205-2213

Chapter 4

Mistreatment of Women in Health Facilities by Midwives during Childbirth in Ghana: Prevalence and Associated Factors

John Kuumuori Ganle and Ebenezer Krampah

Additional information is available at the end of the chapter

http://dx.doi.org/10.5772/intechopen.82432

Abstract

Studies have shown that many women worldwide experience mistreatment during pregnancy and childbirth. However, there are few quantitative estimates of the prevalence of mistreatment of women during facility-based childbirth in many developing countries including Ghana. Based on a cross-sectional retrospective survey of 253 randomly selected women who gave birth between November 2017 and April 2018 in a second-tier referral hospital in Ghana, this study examines mistreatment of women by midwives during childbirth and associated factors. Bivariate and logistic regression analyses were performed at 95% confidence level and $p < 0.05$. Results show that 83% of women were mistreated. Manifestations of mistreatments included detention for non-payment of bills (43.1%), non-confidential care (39.5%), abandonment (30.8%), verbal abuse (25.3%), discrimination (21.3%), physical abuse (14.2%) and non-consented care (13.3%). Factors that significantly independently predicted mistreatment after potential confounders were controlled for were being HIV positive (aOR: 0.11; 95% CI = 0.022–0.608; $p = 0.011$), being attended by a midwife rather than an obstetrician/gyneacologist (aOR: 0.07; 95% CI = 0.018–0.279; $p < 0.01$), and a woman's husband earning lower monthly income. There is need for interventions to train midwives and other maternity care service providers in patient-centered care and interpersonal communication so as to minimize mistreatment of women during childbirth.

Keywords: mistreatment, pregnancy and childbirth, respectful maternal care, midwives, Ghana

1. Introduction

Worldwide, a growing body of research suggests that, many women experience poor treatment during childbirth [1–4]. While the WHO [5] continues to emphasise that every woman has the right to the highest attainable standard of health, which includes the right to dignified and respectful healthcare, many women are reported to experience disrespectful and abusive treatment during pregnancy and childbirth in health facilities worldwide [1–4]. Such mistreatment includes physical abuse, non-consented care, non-confidential care, non-dignified care including verbal abuse, discrimination based on specific attributes, abandonment of care and detention in health facilities [1–4].

Mistreatment of women in health facilities during childbirth is particularly worse in many low-income countries in Africa [6, 7]. For instance, a recent study showed that the prevalence of any form of mistreatment in an exit survey among a sample of 641 women who recently delivered in healthcare facilities in Kenya was 20% [8]. Another study revealed that 15% of women who delivered in a referral hospital in Tanzania reported experiencing one or more forms of abusive and disrespectful care, and this proportion reached to 78% among women who delivered in healthcare facilities in Ethiopia [2]. A systematic review also mentions in southeastern Nigeria that mistreatment of women in a teaching hospital was almost universal such that all of the women reported at least one kind of mistreatment during childbirth [9]. Women commonly reported physical abuse (35.7%), including being "restrained or tied down during labour" (17.3%) and being "beaten, slapped, or pinched" (7.2%); while being "sexually abused by a health worker" was reported by 2.0% of the women [9]. Similarly, a qualitative study exploring mistreatment of women in rural Tanzania estimated that 19.5% of women who reported experiencing any form of mistreatment during childbirth in the facility increased to 28.2% during a follow up survey of same women within 5–10 weeks postpartum [10]. Some 18.9% of the women reported receiving non-dignified care; 13.8% reported being abused verbally; 15.5% reported being neglected; and 5.1% reported being abused physically [10]. In Ghana, previous qualitative research has also documented that mistreatment during facility-based delivery is a salient issue, that sometimes prevent women from seeking skilled birth services [4, 11, 12].

Given the potential for mistreatment during childbirth to undermine future use of skilled birth services in health facilities, the WHO [5] has called for greater research, action, advocacy and dialogue on this important public health issue, in order to ensure safe, timely, and respectful care during childbirth for all women. Likewise, respectful care is a key component of both the mother-baby friendly birth facility initiative currently being implemented in many low-income settings, and the WHO's vision for quality of care for childbearing women and newborns [5]. To date, however, there have been few quantitative estimates of the prevalence of mistreatment of women during facility-based childbirth in Ghana and the determinants of such mistreatment [4, 13]. This knowledge gap could potentially hamper efforts to ensure that all women receive respectful and dignified care during pregnancy and childbirth in Ghana.

http://dx.doi.org/10.5772/intechopen.82432

The study reported in this chapter was therefore undertaken to respond to the WHO's call for greater research on the topic of mistreatment of women during childbirth. Specifically, the objective was to determine the prevalence and forms of mistreatment of women by midwives during childbirth and associated factors. Results, which are presented and discussed below, suggest that mistreatment of childbearing women in health facilities is indeed an important issue in contemporary midwifery and nursing care in Ghana that needs to be urgently addressed.

The rest of the chapter proceeds as follows. The empirical research methods are next described. Results are then presented, followed by a discussion of the results. The final section concludes with some recommendations.

2. Materials and methods

2.1. Study design

A health facility-based retrospective cross-sectional quantitative survey was conducted. Validated survey questionnaires were used to collect data to estimate the prevalence of mistreatments women received during their most recent childbirth, and also determine the association between various exposure variables and the outcome of interest—mistreatment.

2.2. Study setting

Empirical research was conducted in Ghana, a low-income country in West Africa. Ghana is one of the countries in Africa where maternal mortality remains a challenge. For instance, out of 5247 deaths among women aged 15–49 in 2014, 12.1% (634) were pregnancy-related [4]. Low levels of health facility delivery are partly responsible for this relatively high number of maternal deaths [11, 12]. Recent data suggest that out of 794,000 live births annually in Ghana, only 76% are attended by skilled professionals [14]. Despite the fact that the Government of Ghana has implemented initiatives to increase facility-based delivery, including making antenatal care and skilled delivery free [15], giving special attention to pregnant women to easily complete the processes of the National Health Insurance Scheme (NHIS) registration and waiving enrolment fees into the NHIS, as well as scaling up safe motherhood and child survival interventions [16], many women in Ghana still give birth outside health facilities without skilled care [14]. Recent studies have suggested poor quality of maternal healthcare services and mistreatment of women as key reasons why some women in Ghana do not deliver in health facilities [4, 11, 12].

Within Ghana, empirical data collection took place in the Tema General Hospital in the Tema Metropolis of the Greater Accra region. The population of the Tema Metropolis, according to the 2010 Population and Housing Census, is 292,773, representing 7.3% of the region's total population [17]. Females represent 52.2% of the total population of the metropolis. Also, nearly all of the population in the metropolis lives in urban localities [17]. The Metropolis has five government health facilities, 58 private health facilities, four quasi-government facilities and 32 community-based health planning and services (CHPS) zones [18]. The Tema General Hospital serves as the main referral Hospital in the Metropolis with regard to maternal healthcare for both private and public health facilities [18]. This is the main reason why it was chosen for this study. The maternity block of the Hospital has a total of 294-bed capacity [18]. The facility recorded 7000 deliveries in the year 2016, of which 2035 were deliveries by caesarean section and 41 maternal deaths [18].

2.3. Study population

The study's population comprised all women who had given birth at the Tema General Hospital between November 2017 and April, 2018. However, women who had complicated births as well as women who had stillbirths were excluded. We excluded these categories of women because complicated or stillbirths may typically require additionally invasive interventions which could unduly affect women's judgement about mistreatment. Besides, women who go through complicated birth or stillbirth may experience physical and emotional stress, which could also affect their judgement about mistreatment during childbirth.

2.4. Sample size estimation

A minimum sample size of 230 was first estimated using Cochran's statistical formula for cross-sectional studies [19]. The sample size estimation was based on the following assumptions:

1. Confidence level was set at 95%.
2. Prevalence of mistreatment of women in the sample was assumed to be 20%. This assumption was based on a recent study in Kenya which found overall prevalence of mistreatment to be 20% [8].
3. Margin of error (5% = 0.05).

The minimum sample size of 230 was adjusted upward by 10% to cater for possible incompleteness of data. Thus, the final sample size for the study was 253.

2.5. Sampling procedure

A simple random sampling method was used to select the 253 respondents. To ensure that each qualified potential respondent in the sampling frame had equal chance of being included in the study, the register of all women who had given birth in the facility between November 2017 and April, 2018 and were attending child welfare clinic (CWC) at the Tema General Hospital was obtained from the senior nursing officer of the maternity unit. Using the inclusion and exclusion criteria outlined above, the names of all women who had live and uncomplicated births were compiled in excel spreadsheet. In all, a total of 2357 potentially qualified women were identified. Each of the 2357 women was then given a unique number, starting from 0001 to the last woman on the list i.e. 2357. The numbered list was then exported into a Google-based random number generator software and the 253 respondents were randomly selected. Following this selection, a visit was made to the CWC of the Tema General Hospital to meet each selected woman on the day she was scheduled to attend the CWC. During this meeting, we explained the purpose of the study to selected women as well as how they were selected. The women were then given time (2 weeks) to decide their participation. After the 2 weeks, each woman was contacted via telephone. Where the decision was in favour of participation, a date and interview venue were agreed upon between the authors and each woman. Most women agreed to do the interview during their next visit to the CWC, which happened between May and July 2018. However, for any selected woman who did not come to the CWC in the course of the study (there were 3 such cases) or opted not to take part in the study (there were 4 such cases), such women were replaced by repeating the random selection process on the remainder of the women not selected in previous round/s of random selection.

2.6. Data collection methods and instruments

Data was collected through face-to-face survey from May to July, 2018. A structured, closed-ended questionnaire was designed for the data collection. The questionnaire focused on collecting information on a number of issues including socio-demographic characteristics, reproductive and maternal health history, and experiences of mistreatment during childbirth. We adopted and adapted several validated questions from previous researchers [1–3, 8, 20, 21], based on Bowser and Hill's [22] typology of mistreatment. Our operational definitions of the specific components of mistreatment we were interested in are summarised in **Table 1**. The questionnaires were in English, but were asked in English and three other local dialects (*Ga*, *Twi*, and *Ewe*) depending on which one a respondent was fluent in. The second author who collected the data speaks all three local dialects fluently.

Category of mistreatment	Example
Physical abuse	Hitting, roughly forcing legs apart for delivery
Non-consented care	No informed consent for procedures, such as when provider elects to perform unnecessary episiotomy
Non-confidential care	No privacy (spatial, visual, or auditory)
Non-dignified care	Humiliation by shouting, blaming, or degrading
Discrimination based on specific patient attributes	HIV status, ethnicity, age, marital status, language, economic status, educational level, etc.
Abandonment of care	Facility closed despite being 24/7, or if open, no staff can or do attend delivery
Detention in facilities	Not releasing mother until bill is paid

Table 1. Type and definition of mistreatment.

2.7. Pre-test and quality assurance

The questionnaires were pre-tested in the CWC of another public health facility in the Tema Metropolis using 20 randomly selected mothers who gave birth between November 2017 and April 2018. The pretest enabled ambiguities in the wording of some questions to be corrected. The pretest also enabled us estimate the average time required to complete each questionnaire. In addition to the pretesting, other quality assurance measures were implemented. Data collected by the second author were checked every day by the first author to ensure accuracy and completeness. Errors that were detected were discussed and where needed, follow up interviews were made to correct any such errors.

2.8. Data processing and analysis

2.8.1. Data entry and processing

The completed questionnaires were hand-coded and entered into Microsoft Excel. The data were then exported to Stata 15 version software for further cleaning. Cleaning of the data was done by running frequencies on each variable. This checked inconsistently coded data. Inconsistently coded data were double checked with raw data from the questionnaire, and all inconsistencies and errors were resolved.

2.8.2. Variables

The dependent variable in this study is mistreatment of women during childbirth. Mistreatment was defined as specific behaviours of providers, which are related to any of the seven categories of mistreatment listed in **Table 1**, and expressed towards mothers in ways that are disrespectful or humiliating [23]. Questions on mistreatments were measured as dichotomous, such that any respondent who reported experiencing any of the seven categories of mistreatment in **Table 1** was considered mistreated.

A number of independent variables expected to influence mistreatment were also measured. These included socio-demographic characteristics such as age, marital status, income level, educational level and religion. Other maternal and health system factors included mode of delivery, type of birth attendant, HIV status and antenatal care (ANC) attendance during pregnancy.

2.8.3. Statistical analysis

Descriptive statistical analysis (frequency, mean and standard deviation) was performed to describe important characteristics of respondents as well as estimate prevalence and forms of mistreatment women received during childbirth. Bivariate and logistic regression analyses were then performed to examine factors associated with mistreatment of women during childbirth. Statistical significance was considered at 95% confidence level and a $p < 0.05$.

2.9. Ethical issues

Ethical approval was sought and obtained from the Ghana Health Service Ethical Review Committee. In addition, administrative consent and approval to conduct the study in the hospital was sought and obtained from the director of medical services of the Tema General

http://dx.doi.org/10.5772/intechopen.82432

Hospital. Participation in the study was entirely voluntary, and this was communicated to all selected respondents. Before interviews were conducted, each participant signed or thumb printed an informed consent form to confirm their voluntary consent to participate in the study. However, respondents were told that they could withdraw consent and discontinue their participation in the study without any adverse consequences. Also, as some aspects of the mistreatment some women received were emotionally traumatising for them to recount during our study, we ensured that all such women were referred to a clinical psychologist based at the same health facility for counselling. However, this process was entirely voluntary, and no woman was referred if she did not want to see the psychologist. In addition, interviews were conducted in a private room where maximum anonymity and confidentiality were ensured. No direct compensation or benefits were paid to respondents. However, each respondent received age and sex-appropriate toy for their baby worth only GH₵5 ($1).

3. Results

3.1. Socio-demographic characteristics of respondents

Questionnaires were successfully completed for all the 253 respondents. **Table 2** shows the background characteristics of respondents. The mean age was 28.1 years (SD = ± 6.0). The majority (34.4%) were aged 24–29 years. The majority (32.4%) also attained secondary school education, while only 9.9% had no formal education. Also, 69.6% were heterosexually married, and most marriages (65.7%) were monogamous. Christians were in the majority (87.4%). In terms of parity, majority (86.2%) of the respondents had between 1 and 3 children.

Characteristics	Frequency	Percent (%)
Age		
15–19	13	5.15
20–24	63	24.90
25–29	87	34.39
30–34	49	19.37
35–39	26	10.28
40–44	15	5.93
Level of education		
No formal education	25	9.88
Primary	36	14.23
JHS	81	32.02
Secondary	82	32.41
Tertiary	29	11.46
Marital status		
Married	176	69.57
Separated	14	5.53

Characteristics	Frequency	Percent (%)
Co-habiting	28	11.07
Single	35	13.83
Type of marriage		
Monogamous	134	65.69
Polygamous	70	34.31
Religious affiliation		
Christianity	221	87.35
Islamic	29	11.46
Traditional	3	1.19
Residence		
Urban	241	95.26
Rural	12	4.74
Ethnicity		
Ga	54	21.43
Twi	56	22.22
Fante	36	14.29
Ewe	47	18.65
Others	59	23.41
Occupation		
Trading	100	39.53
Housewife	53	20.95
Seamstress	28	11.07
Hairdresser	23	9.09
Civil servants	25	9.88
Others	24	9.49
Monthly income (GH₵)		
No salary	57	22.53
<GHc500	165	65.22
GHc500–1000	22	8.70
>GHc1000	9	3.56
Parity		
1–3 children	218	86.17
4–7 children	35	13.83
Dependents		
1–3 dependants	169	85.79

http://dx.doi.org/10.5772/intechopen.82432

Characteristics	Frequency	Percent (%)
4–7 dependants	28	14.21
Husbands' level of education		
No formal education	17	6.85
Primary	17	6.86
JHS	62	25.00
Secondary	99	39.92
Tertiary	53	21.37
Husband's occupation		
None	21	8.30
Trading	49	19.37
Civil servant	39	15.42
Farmer	16	6.32
Others	128	50.59
Husband's monthly income (GH₵)		
100–500	111	50.45
500–1000	77	35.00
1000–1500	21	9.55
2000–2500	11	5.00

Table 2. Socio-demographic characteristics.

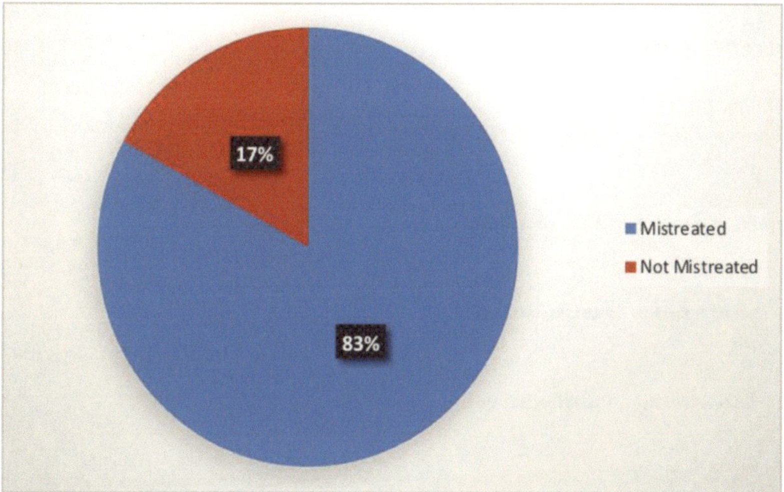

Figure 1. Prevalence of mistreatment.

3.2. Prevalence of mistreatment

Figure 1 summarises the prevalence of mistreatment among the women surveyed. The overall prevalence of mistreatment was 83.0%. This included those who suffered at least one form of mistreatment in the facility during their most recent childbirth. The most common form of mistreatment was detention for long hours for non-payment of medical bills (43.1%), followed by non-confidential care (39.5%), abandonment (30.8%), verbal abuse (25.3%), discrimination (21.3%) and physical abuse (14.2%) (see **Table 3**).

Types of mistreatments	Description	Response	
		Yes (%)	No (%)
Physical abuse (n=253)	Hitting, beating, slapping, pitching, legs held.	36(14.2)	217(85.8)
Verbal abuse/Non-dignified (n=153)	Shouted at, reprimanded, insult.	64(25.3)	89(74.7)
Non-Confidential (n=253)	No privacy (spatial, visual, or auditory)	100(39.5)	53(60.47)
Non-Consented (n=240)	No informed consent for procedures, such as episiotomy, HIV status.	32(13.3)	208(86.67)
Discrimination (n=253)	Age, marital status, inadequate preparation, financial status.	54(21.3)	199(78.7)
Detention (n=253)	Not releasing mother until bill is paid.	109(43.1)	144(56.92)
Abandonment (n=244)	Leaving women to deliver alone, no help from providers after Cs	76(31.9)	168(68.9)

Table 3. Types of mistreatment women received.

Multiple experience of mistreatment	Frequency	Percent (%)
Experienced 2 forms of mistreatment		
Yes	65	25.69
No	188	74.31
Experienced 3 forms of mistreatment		
Yes	44	17.39
No	209	82.61
Experienced 4 forms of mistreatment		
Yes	28	11.07
No	225	88.93
Experienced 5 forms of mistreatment		
Yes	14	5.53
No	239	94.47
Experienced 6 forms of mistreatment		
Yes	1	0.83
No	252	99.60
Experienced 7 forms of mistreatment		
Yes	0	0
No	253	100

Table 4. Multiple experiences of mistreatments.

Characteristics	Mistreated		
	Yes	No	Chi-square P-value
Age			
15–19	7(58.33)	5(41.67)	0.046*
20–24	58(92.06)	5(7.94)	
25–29	74(85.06)	13(14.94)	
30–34	36(73.47)	13(26.53)	
35–39	19(73.08)	7(26.92)	
40–44	10(66.67)	5(33.33)	
Marital status			
Married	140(79.55)	36(20.45)	0.205
Separated	9(64.29)	5(35.71)	
Co-habiting	20(74.43)	8(28.57)	
Single	30(85.71)	5(14.29)	
Type of marriage			
Monogamous	105(78.36)	29(21.64)	0.072
Polygamous	62 (88.57)	8(11.43)	
Level of education			
No formal education	20(80.00)	5(20.00)	0.048*
Primary	72(88.89)	9(11.11)	
JHS	30(83.33)	6(16.67)	
Secondary	65(79.27)	17(20.73)	
Tertiary	19(65.52)	10(34.48)	
Residence			
Urban	198(82.16)	43(17.84)	0.228
Rural	7(58.33)	5(41.67)	
Religious affiliation			
Christianity	181(81.10)	40(18.10)	0.677
Islamic	22 (75.86)	7(24.14)	
Traditional	6(54.55.00)	5(45.45)	
Occupation			
Trading	85(85.00)	15(17.0)	0.384
Housewife	46(86.79)	7(13.21)	
Seamstress	22(78.57)	6(21.43)	

Characteristics	Mistreated		
	Yes	No	Chi-square P-value
Hairdresser	17(73.91)	6(26.09)	
Civil servants	17(68.00)	8(32.00)	
Others	18(75.00)	6(25.00)	
Monthly income (GH₵)			
No salary	51(89.47)	6(10.53)	0.045*
<GHc500	138(83.64)	27(16.36)	
GHc500–1000	16(72.73)	6(27.27)	
>GHc1000	6(54.55)	5(45.45)	
Ethnicity			
Ga	44(81.48)	10(18.52)	0.849
Twi	46(82.14)	10(17.86)	
Fante	29(80.56)	7(19.44)	
Ewe	39(82.98)	8(17.02)	
Others	52(88.14)	7(11.86)	
Parity			
1–3 children	180(82.57)	38(17.43)	0.646
4–7 children	30(85.71)	5(14.29)	
Dependents			
1–3 dependants	138(81.66)	31(18.34)	0.425
4–7 dependants	21(75.00)	7(25.00)	
Husbands' level of education			
No formal education	11(64.71)	6(35.29)	0.056
Primary	11(64.71)	6(35.29)	
JHS	57(91.94)	5(8.06)	
Secondary	77(77.47)	22(22.22)	
Tertiary	40(75.47)	13(24.53)	
Husband's occupation			
None	14(66.67).	7(33.33)	0.151
Trading	43(87.76)	6(12.24)	
Civil servant	30(76.92)	9(23.08)	
Farmer	10(62.50)	6(37.50)	
Others	103(80.47)	25(19.53)	

Characteristics	Mistreated		
	Yes	No	Chi-square P-value
Husband's monthly income (GH₵)			
100–500	97(87.39)	14(12.61)	0.002*
500–1000	64(83.12)	13(16.88)	
1000–1500	12(57.14)	9(42.86)	
2000–2500	6(54.55)	5(45.45)	

Table 5. Socio-demographic factors associated with mistreatments (bivariate analyses). *$p < 0.05$

Characteristics	Mistreated		
	Yes	No	Chi-square P-value
ANC attendance			
Yes	201(84.10)	38(15.90)	1.000
No	9(62.29)	5(35.71)	
Age of the baby (n = 200)			
1–3 months and below	120(85.71)	20(14.29)	0.201
4–6 months	90(79.65)	23(20.35)	
Mode of delivery			
Vaginal delivery	141(85.98)	23(14.02)	0.088
Caesarean section	69(77.53)	20(22.47)	
Birth attendant			
Obstetrician/gyneacologist	64(77.11)	19(22.89)	0.000*
Midwife	146(85.88)	24(14.12)	
HIV status			
Negative	151(95.32)	9(4.68)	0.009*
Positive	73(78.49)	20(21.51)	
Had episiotomy			
Yes	193(83.55)	38(16.45)	1.000
No	6(54.55)	5(45.45)	
Had a bed			
Yes	202(84.17)	38(15.83)	0.220
No	8(61.54)	5(38.46)	

Table 6. Maternal and health system factors associated with mistreatment (bivariate analyses). *$p < 0.05$

As shown in **Table 4**, many women experienced multiple forms of mistreatment during their most recent health facility delivery. The majority of women (25.7%) suffered from two types of mistreatment; 17.4% suffered three types of mistreatment; 11.1% suffered four different types of mistreatment; and 5.5% suffered five types of mistreatment. Only 0.8% of the women suffered six types of mistreatment, with no respondent reporting suffering all the seven types of mistreatment studied.

3.3. Factors associated with mistreatment

Table 5 presents information on bivariate analysis investigating the association between socio-demographic factors and mistreatment based on chi-square test of independence. Age of mother (p = 0.046), mother's level of education (p = 0.048), mother's monthly income (p = 0.045), and husband's monthly income (p = 0.002) were statistically significantly associated with mistreatment of women during their most recent childbirth in the Tema General Hospital. In addition to the socio-demographic factors, other maternal and health system factors were assessed. The results are shown in **Table 6**. A woman's HIV status (p = 0.009), as well as type of birth attendant during childbirth (p < 0.01) were statistically associated with mistreatment.

In total, six (6) factors showed statistical association with mistreatment at the bivariate level. These were pulled into a logistic regression model in a second round of analysis. A simple logistic regression analyses model, followed by a multiple logistic regression analyses model, were then performed on the six variables. The results are shown in **Table 7**. After adjusting

Characteristics	Mistreated Yes	Mistreated No	Unadjusted OR (95%CI)	P-value	Adjusted OR (95%CI)	P-value
Age						
15-19 *(ref)*	7(58.33)	5(41.67)				
20-24	58(92.06)	5(7.94)	0.97(0.103-9.037)	0.976	0.97(0.1034-9.037)	0.976
25-29	74(85.06)	13(14.94)	0.47(0.057-3.966)	0.491	0.47(0.057-3.966)	0.491
30-34	36(73.47)	13(26.53)	0.23(0.027-1.954)	0.179	0.23(0.027-1.954)	0.179
35-39	19(73.08)	7(26.92)	0.25(0.025-2.075)	0.189	0.23(0.025-2.075)	0.189
40-44	10(66.67)	5(33.33)	0.23(0.022-2.377)	0.217	0 23(0.022-2377)	0.217
Level of Education						
No Formal Education *(ref)*	20(80.00)	5(20.00)				
Primary	72(88.89)	9(11.11)	1.09(0.222-5.362)	0.915	0.48(0.551-4.216)	0.509
JHS	30(83.33)	6(16.67)	1.09(0.271-4.385)	0.902	0.90(0.145-5.600)	
0.910						
Secondary	65(79.27)	17(20.73)	0.52(0.139-1.950)	0.333	0.37(0.061-2.238)	0.278
Tertiary	19(65.52)	10(34.48)	0.26(0.062-1.081)	0.064	0.41(0.042-4.045)	0.446
Mother's monthly income (GHȻ)						
No salary *(ref)*	51(89.47)	6(10.53)				
<GHc500	138(83.64)	27(16.36)	0.60(0.235-1.541)	0.289	0.57(0.162-2.024)	0.386
GHc500-1000	16(72.73)	6(27.27)	0.31(0.089-1.110)	0.072	0.80(0.125-5.147)	0.816
>GHc1000	5(55.56)	4(44.44)	0.15(0.031-0.702)*	0.016	0.39(0.034-4.886)	0.462
Husband's monthly income (GHȻ)						
100-500 *(ref)*	97(87.39)	14(12.61)				
500-1000	64(83.12)	13(16.88)	0.71(0.313-1.610)	0.413	0.53(0.1907-1.457)	0.217
1000-1500	12(57.14)	9(42.86)	0.19(0.069-0.539)*	0.002	0.19(0.041-0.883)*	0.034*
2000-2500	6(54.55)	5(45.45)	0.18(0.043-0.753)*	0.019	0.33(0.042-2.424)	0.274
HIV Status						
Positive *(ref)*	53(56.99)	40(43.01)				
Negative	151(95.32)	9(4.68)	0.22(0.065-0.746)*	0.015	0.11(0.022-0.608)*	0.011*
Birth Attendant						
Midwife *(ref)*	146(85.88)	24(14.12)				
Obstetrician/gyneacologist	64 (77.11)	19(22.89)	0.09(0.026-0.291)*	0.000	0.07(0.018-0.279)	0.000*

Table 7. Predictors of mistreatment during childbirth (logistic regression analysis). *p < 0.05

for potential confounders, husband's income, HIV status and type of birth attendant during childbirth independently predicted mistreatment. Specifically, the odds of being mistreated were significantly lower for HIV negative women compared to HIV positive women (cOR: 0.22; 95% CI = 0.065–0.746; p = 0.015). This relationship was still statistically significant after potential confounders were adjusted for (aOR: 0.11; 95% CI = 0.022–0.608; p = 0.011). Women whose births were attended by obstetricians/gyneacologists were also significantly less likely to report mistreatment compared to those whose birth were attended by midwives (cOR: 0.09; 95% CI = 0.026–0.291; p < 0.01). This relationship was still strongly statistically significant after other factors were adjusted for (aOR: 0.07; 95% CI = 0.018–0.279; p < 0.01). Also, as a woman's husband's monthly income increases, the odds of the woman reporting mistreatment reduces, although the relationship was generally very weak.

4. Discussion

This study is among the first in Ghana to quantitatively estimate the prevalence of mistreatment of women during health facility-based childbirth and associated factors. Findings suggest that, the overall prevalence of mistreatment of women during their most recent childbirth in the Tema General Hospital was high (83%), with most of the mothers experiencing detention (43.1%) due to lack of fee payment, non-confidential care (39.5%), neglect/abandonment (31.8%), verbal abuse (25.3%), discrimination (21.3%), physical abuse (14.2%), and non-consented care (13.3%). Many women also experienced multiple forms of mistreatment. The main factors that significantly predicted mistreatment were being HIV positive, being attended by a midwife rather than an obstetrician/gyneacologist, and a woman's husband earning lower monthly income.

A number of our findings above deserves further commentary. Compared to other previous studies in Africa [8, 9], the 83% prevalence of mistreatment in this study is relatively high. It is however not surprising as evidence from a recent systematic review suggests that mistreatment is increasing in many low-income settings especially in urban areas [13]. With increasing population in many urban areas in SSA amid declining human and financial resources for health as well as deteriorating health infrastructure, there are suggestions that congestion in maternity wards, under-staffing, and over working of health staff, may be compromising quality of maternity care, including mistreatment of women during childbirth [21, 24–26]. It is also possible that mistreatment may not be increasing per se; just that many urban women are becoming increasingly aware of their rights as patients partly because of improvements in formal education. This is more likely in the present study given that the majority of women had some formal education. Be that as it may, the relatively high prevalence of mistreatment in this study is a cause for concern. Mistreatment of women in health facilities during childbirth does not only violate the rights of women to respectful care, but can also threaten women's rights to life, health, bodily integrity, and freedom from institutional violence [5]. Thus, not only is mistreatment a public health issue but it also becomes a human rights and an equity issue [10]. As a number of studies have shown, women who experience mistreatment from midwives or other maternity care providers in a health facility setting are often less likely to go to a health facility again in subsequent childbirth [4, 11, 12]. This suggests a need for interventions to raise awareness among maternity care providers about the potential adverse effect mistreatment of women could have on utilisation of skilled birth services in the future, and the need to treat women with respect and dignity during childbirth.

This study also indicated that 43% of women who were detained after delivery were as a result of non-payment of medical bills. This is an important factor especially in SSA where women are not as economically empowered as men, and one would therefore expect to find many women with very low monthly income. This seems to be the case in this study where women appeared to earn far lower monthly incomes than their husbands, and where husbands' monthly income was a significant determinant of mistreatment. Indeed, in an Ethiopian study, women with higher monthly incomes were less likely to experience mistreatment as compared to those with a lower monthly income [7]. In countries that still have a user-fee system, poor women may be detained in hospitals after delivery for failure to pay the required bills. A recent study in Ghana indicated that 22% of the women in the sample were detained in health facilities after delivery for nonpayment of fees [9]. Our finding in relation to the relatively high detention rate of women after birth is however surprising given that Ghana has since 2005 implemented a user-fee exemption policy for skilled delivery services. It could be the case that there are other informal charges not covered under the user-fee exemption policy. This is more likely given that previous research in Ghana has reported the existence of informal charges in many health facilities despite the existence of the NHIS and the user-fee exemption policy for delivery services. Our findings here would suggest a need to relook at the user-fee exemption policy for maternal healthcare services to ensure that services are truly free for women. Also, ensuring timely enrolment of all pregnant women on the NHIS through the user-fee exemption policy could lessen the financial burden mothers and families may go through during childbirth.

Again, non-consented care (no informed consent before procedures), non-confidential care, performing vaginal examination in the presence of other people, including patients, as well as disclosure of medical history without consent were other forms of mistreatment mothers went through during delivery. These findings could be due to under-staffing, lack of resources and smaller size of the labour ward and delivery rooms in the hospital. The findings here imply that, expanding the staffing numbers and labour ward and partitioning the rooms with low-cost curtains may have a great bearing on ensuring privacy and respectful maternity care.

Another important finding relates to the fact that women who were HIV positive were more likely to report being mistreated compared to those who were HIV negative. This is not so surprising given that HIV/AIDS is still largely a highly moralising and stigmatising disease in many contexts in Africa. Our result here however does suggest a need for maternity care providers to be less judgmental and discriminatory when dealing with HIV positive mothers. Rather, compassionate and dignified care needs to be emphasised in the care delivery process.

Finally, women whose births were attended by obstetricians/gyneacologists were also significantly less likely to report mistreatment compared to those whose births were attended by midwives. Given that majority of births in this study, and indeed in most parts of Ghana and SSA are attended by midwives, our finding here is very concerning. Lack of cultural competency, limited training on patient-centred care as well as low staffing numbers and work overload among midwives are possible factors that could contribute to midwives inadvertently mistreating women during childbirth. This would again suggest a need to further strengthen the core training curriculum of midwives to emphasise patient-centred care and interpersonal communication and relationships in addition to increasing the staffing numbers and expanding infrastructure to enhance the interaction between midwives and women during childbirth. Regular on-the-job training of midwives to improve the cultural competency skills alongside improved supervision and greater accountability in the labour wards could all help lessen mistreatment.

Although findings from this study would provide useful information that could guide policy and practice to reduce mistreatment of women in health facilities during childbirth, the study has some limitations. A major limitation is the cross-sectional retrospective survey design that was used, which did not offer opportunities for observational and longitudinal analysis to be done. Observing the interactions between women and maternity care givers would particularly have provided important nuances and as well introduce validation mechanisms into the data collection process. Also, there could be recall bias as respondents were made to recall events that happened in the past 6 months prior to this study. These limitations aside, we believe important lessons could be learnt from our study. Also, our findings could form the basis for a large-scale, more elaborate study using both qualitative and quantitative methods along with health facility audits, to determine the scale of mistreatment of women during childbirth in both urban and rural health facility contexts, and the drivers of mistreatment.

5. Conclusion

This study aimed to examine the prevalence of mistreatment of women during childbirth in health facilities in Ghana, and the factors associated with such mistreatment. Results revealed the prevalence (83%) of mistreatment of women during childbirth in the Tema General Hospital to be high. The specific types of mistreatments varied from woman to woman, but the most prevalent forms were detention, physical mistreatment (hitting, slapping, pinching, legs held and forced apart), and verbal abuse (shouted at, insulted, and reprimanded). A number of factors have been identified to be statistically related to mistreatment, including husbands' monthly income, being HIV positive, and being attended in childbirth by a midwife as against an obstetrician/gynaecologist.

Taken together, the results and discussions in this study add to a growing body of evidence across Africa including in Nigeria [1], Tunisia [2], Ethiopia [7, 20, 25], Kenya [8, 24], and Guinea [21] that suggests mistreatment of women during childbirth as an important public health and human rights issue. Our study, together with evidence from previous research within Africa, gives an indication of the factors that may be contributing to mistreatment of women during childbirth. We think the widespread nature of the phenomena of mistreatment of women thus far in many countries in Africa has clear implications for midwifery and future research. First, we think our findings provide a basis for large-scale further quantitative and qualitative studies in different contexts in Ghana and in other African countries to estimate the prevalence and forms of mistreatment of women during childbirth, identify important determinants, and explore detailed contextual, structural and personal level explanatory factors as well as relevant remedial policy options and interventions. Second, and beyond this proposed research agenda, we think the time has come for this evidence to be taken up more seriously not just by individual countries like Ghana or health facilities like the Tema General Hospital, but also by midwifery training institutions and professional bodies in different African countries such as the Ghana College of Nurses and Midwives and the West African College of Nurses and Midwives. In addition to a need for critical self-reflection and professional re-orientation of the practice of contemporary nursing and midwifery care within these training institutions and professional organisations to uphold human rights and patient dignity, there should also be professional ethics training for midwives as part of both the core curriculum for training midwives and routine in-service or on-the-job training. This training could also include patient-centred care and interpersonal communication and relationships building.

Given that women who experience mistreatments from healthcare providers are less likely to go to the health facility again during future pregnancy and childbirth, our results also have specific practical implications for the Ghana Health Service more generally, and the Tema General Hospital more specifically. It is important that interventions are put in place to train service providers in patient-centred care and interpersonal communication and relationships so as to minimise mistreatment. Specifically, the Tema General Hospital, together with the Ghana Health Service (GHS), and the Ministry of Health (MoH) should strengthen education of both patients and healthcare providers on patients' rights and responsibilities under the Patients' Charter, and to establish reporting mechanisms in the hospital so that women who suffer unjust mistreatments during childbirth could feel free to report and be responded to appropriately. A sanctions regime, including temporary suspension and total dismissal from work, should also be considered in this regard to deter healthcare providers who unjustifiably mistreat women. Before the above recommendations are implemented however, we recommend expansion in health infrastructure especially in urban areas as well as increasing the human resource base especially the number of midwives so as to reduce work overload and overwork. Finally, there is a need for both public and private sector health facilities that provide maternity care to women to liaise with the GHS and the MoH to ensure that the free maternal health benefit package under the NHIS is comprehensive and covers all women in order to eliminate all informal payments. Also, sanctions should be meted out to healthcare providers who charge unofficial fees. This could help reduce the phenomenon of maternity detention after birth, which contributes to mistreatment.

Acknowledgements

This manuscript was first drafted when the first author (JKG) was a Fellow at the Stellenbosch Institute for Advanced Study (STIAS), Stellenbosch University, South Africa. Writing space for the manuscript was graciously provided by STIAS. We are grateful for this support.

Conflict of interest

The authors declare that they have no conflict of interest.

Author details

John Kuumuori Ganle[1,2]* and Ebenezer Krampah[1]

*Address all correspondence to: jganle@ug.edu.gh

1 Department of Population, Family and Reproductive Health, School of Public Health, University of Ghana, Accra, Ghana

2 Stellenbosch Institute for Advanced Study, Stellenbosch University, South Africa

References

[1] Bohren AM, Vogel PJ, Tunçalp Ö, Fawole B, Titiloye AM, Olutayo OA, et al. "By slapping their laps, the patient will know that you truly care for her": A qualitative study on social norms and acceptability of the mistreatment of women during childbirth in Abuja, Nigeria. SSM-Population Health. 2016;**2**:640-655. DOI: 10.1016/j.ssmph.2016.07.003

[2] Amroussia N, Hernandez A, Vives-Cases C, Goicolea I. "Is the doctor god to punish me?!" An intersectional examination of disrespectful and abusive care during childbirth against single mothers in Tunisia. Reproductive Health. 2017;**14**(1):1-12. DOI: 10.1186/s12978-017-0290-9

[3] Diamond-Smith N, Sudhinaraset M, Melo J, Murthy N. The relationship between women's experiences of mistreatment at facilities during childbirth, types of support received and person providing the support in Lucknow, India. Midwifery. 2016;**40**:114-123. DOI: 10.1016/j.midw.2016.06.014

[4] Moyer CA, Adongo PB, Aborigo RA, Hodgson A, Engmann CM. "They treat you like you are not a human being": Maltreatment during labour and delivery in rural northern Ghana. Midwifery. 2014;**30**(2):262-268. DOI: 10.1016/j.midw.2013.05.006

[5] WHO. The Prevention and Elimination of Disrespect and Abuse during Facility-Based Childbirth. Geneva: World Health Organisation; 2015

[6] Cerón A, Ruano AL, Sánchez S, Chew AS, Díaz D, Hernández A, et al. Abuse and discrimination towards indigenous people in public health care facilities: Experiences from rural Guatemala. International Journal for Equity in Health. 2016;**15**(1):1-7. DOI: 10.1186/s12939-016-0367-z

[7] Asefa A, Bekele D. Status of respectful and non-abusive care during facility- based childbirth in a hospital and health centers in Addis Ababa, Ethiopia. Reprodroductive

Health. 2015;**12**(1):33. Available from: http://www.reproductive-health-journal.com/content/12/1/33

[8] Abuya T, Warren CE, Miller N, Njuki R, Ndwiga C, Maranga A, et al. Exploring the prevalence of disrespect and abuse during childbirth in Kenya. PLoS One. 2015;**10**(4):e0123606. DOI: 10.1371/journal.pone.0123606

[9] Ishola F, Owolabi O, Filippi V. Disrespect and abuse of women during childbirth in Nigeria: A systematic review. PLoS One. 2017;**12**(3):e0174084. DOI: 10.1371/journal.pone.0174084

[10] McMahon SA, George AS, Chebet JJ, Mosha IH, Mpembeni RNM, Winch PJ. Experiences of and responses to disrespectful maternity care and abuse during childbirth; a qualitative study with women and men in Morogoro Region, Tanzania. BMC Pregnancy and Childbirth. 2014;**14**(1):1-13. DOI: 10.1186/1471-2393-14-268

[11] Ganle JK, Parker M, Fitpatrick R, Otupiri E. A qualitative study of health system barriers to accessibility and utilization of maternal and newborn healthcare services in Ghana after user-fee abolition. BMC Pregnancy and Childbirth. 2014;**14**:425

[12] Ganle JK, Parker M, Fitpatrick R, Otupiri E. Addressing health system barriers to access to and use of skilled delivery services: Perspectives from Ghana. International Journal of Health Planning and Management. 2015;**31**(4):e235-e253. DOI: 10.1002/hpm.2291

[13] Bohren MA, Vogel JP, Hunter EC, Lutsiv O, Makh SK, Souza JP, et al. The mistreatment of women during childbirth in health facilities globally: A mixed-methods systematic review. PLoS Medicine. 2015;**12**(6):1-32. DOI: 10.1371/journal.pmed.1001847

[14] Ghana Statistical Service (GSS), Ghana Health Service (GHS), ICF. Ghana Maternal Health Survey 2017: Key Indicators Report. Accra, Ghana: GSS, GHS, and ICF; 2018

[15] Ganle JK, Parker M, Fitpatrick R, Otupiri E. Free maternity care and equity of access to maternal health services in Ghana: A descriptive study. International Journal for Equity in Health. 2014;**13**:89

[16] Witter S, Arhinful KD, Kusi A, Zakariah-Akoto S. The experiences of Ghana in implementing a user fee exemption policy to provide free delivery care. Reproductive Health Matters. 2007;**15**(30):61-71

[17] Ghana Statistical Service. Ghana Population and Housing Census 2010. Accra: Ghana Statistical Service; 2012

[18] Ghana Health Service. Annual Health 2016. Accra: Ghana Health Service; 2016

[19] Cohrane WG. Sampling Technique. 3rd ed. New York: John Wiley & Sons; 1977

[20] Burrowes S, Holcombe SJ, Jara D, Carter D, Smith K. Midwives' and patients' perspective on disrespect and abuse during labour and delivery care in Ethiopia: A qualitative study. BMC Pregnancy and Childbirth. 2017;**17**:263. DOI: 10.1186/s12884-017-1442-1

[21] Balde MD, Diallo BA, Bangoura A, Sall O, Soumah AM, Vogel JP, et al. Perceptions and experiences of the mistreatment of women during childbirth in health facilities in

Guinea: A qualitative study with women and service providers. Reproductive Health. 2017;**14**(1):1-13. DOI: 10.1186/s12978-016-0266-1

[22] Bowser D, Hill K. Exploring Evidence for Disrespect and Abuse in Facility- Based Childbirth. Boston: USAID-Tract Project Harvard School Public Health; 2010. Available from: http://www.tractionproject.org/sites/default/files/Respectful_Care_at_Birth_9-20-101_Final.pdf

[23] Freedman LP, Kruk ME. Disrespect and abuse of women in childbirth: Challenging the global quality and accountability agendas. The Lancet. 2014;**384**(9948):e42-e44. DOI: 10.1016/S0140-6736(14)60859-X

[24] Warren CE, Njue R, Ndwiga C, Abuya T. Manifestations and drivers of mistreatment of women during childbirth in Kenya: Implications for measurement and developing interventions. BMC Pregnancy and Childbirth. 2017;**17**(1):1-14. DOI: 10.1186/s12884-017-1288-6

[25] Kruk ME, Paczkowski MM, Tegegn A, et al. Women's preferences for obstetric care in rural Ethiopia: A population-based discrete choice experiment in a region with low rates of facility delivery. Journal of Epidemiology and Community Health. 2010;**64**:984-988

[26] Ratcliffe HL, Sando D, Mwanyika-Sando M, Chalamilla G, Langer A, McDonald KP. Applying a participatory approach to the promotion of a culture of respect during childbirth. Reproductive Health. 2016;**13**(1):1-7. DOI: 10.1186/s12978-016-0186-0

Chapter 5

Improving Maternal Health: The Safe Childbirth Checklist as a Tool for Reducing Maternal Mortality and Morbidity

Julius Dohbit, Vetty Agala, Pamela Chinwa-Banda, Betty Anane-Fenin, Omosivie Maduka, Ufuoma Edewor, Ibimonye Porbeni, Fru Angwafo and Rosemary Ogu

Additional information is available at the end of the chapter

http://dx.doi.org/10.5772/intechopen.82616

Abstract

Ensuring healthy lives and promoting the well-being for all at all ages is essential to sustainable development. The UN's adoption of the sustainable development goals (SDGs) in September 2015 reaffirmed the reduction of maternal and newborn mortality as global priorities in the coming decade. The World Health Organisation Safe Childbirth Checklist has been developed to ensure the delivery of essential maternal and perinatal care practices. The Safe Childbirth Checklist aims to help frontline health workers to prevent avoidable childbirth-related mortality and morbidity. The Checklist addresses the major causes of maternal death (haemorrhage, infection, obstructed labour and hypertensive disorders), intrapartum-related stillbirths (inadequate intrapartum care), and neonatal deaths (birth asphyxia, infection and complications related to prematurity). Successful completion of checklist items by healthcare workers will help keep the woman and baby safe as the checklist catalogues a core set of practices that are proven to reduce maternal and newborn harm. The practices described in the checklist items should be conducted at every birth. This chapter utilises experiences gained in Cameroon, Ghana, Nigeria and Zambia during the Pfizer Independent Grant for Learning and Change supported Medical Women's Association of Nigeria Improving Maternal Health in sub-Saharan Africa project to describe the checklist and how it can be used to deliver lifesaving midwifery care and enhance maternal health.

Keywords: maternal health, safe childbirth checklist, childbirth, safety, quality of care

1. Introduction

The high rate of maternal mortality and morbidity, especially in developing countries calls for international concern. Although the ongoing Sustainable Development Goals (SDGs) has included its prevention as one of the major indicators for measuring global development by the year 2030; success can only ensue if the challenges faced by low-resource settings are recognised and tackled. In about 130 million births per year, an estimated 303,000 result in the mother's death, and 2.6 million in stillbirths [1]. The majority of these deaths, mostly preventable, occur in low-resource settings [2, 3]. The World Health Organisation (WHO) thus developed the Safe Childbirth Checklist to support the delivery of essential birth practices for the prevention of maternal and newborn deaths [4]. The Safe Childbirth Checklist summarises the major direct causes of maternal death such as haemorrhage, hypertensive disorders, infections, and obstructed labour. The Checklist also addresses intrapartum-related stillbirths resulting from inadequate care during labour and delivery and neonatal deaths arising from birth asphyxia, complications related to prematurity, and infections. It was developed from evidence-based birth practices and tested in 10 countries across Asia and Africa [4]. Africa and Asia contribute over 90% of the world's maternal and perinatal deaths.

Childbirth is a complex but physiological process necessitating, sometimes difficult, sometimes complicated steps that prevent adverse outcomes for the mother and her newborn child. Healthcare givers may find it difficult to simply remember all of the relevant information, and performing all the steps perfectly and in the precise order may become challenging especially in the busy labour ward. The WHO Safe Childbirth Checklist is a simple quality improvement tool that reminds healthcare workers to deliver high-quality care from when the woman is admitted, through childbirth, until the woman and baby are safely discharged home.

Checklists prompt users to remember to carry out essential tasks and have long been fundamental to maintaining safety when flying aeroplanes [5]. In other settings, professionals are successfully using checklists to organise large amounts of complex information, to remind themselves to perform crucial duties, and to ultimately do their jobs more effectively and proficiently [5]. In recent years, research on checklists in the health sector has been associated with improved safety with trials of checklist programmes in intensive care medicine and surgery demonstrating significant reductions in complications and deaths [6].

Thus, the WHO, together with obstetricians, paediatricians, nurses, midwives, patient safety experts, developed the WHO Safe Childbirth Checklist and an implementation guide [4] to help healthcare workers improve adherence to proven maternal and newborn care practices. Identifying effective methods to save lives at birth is a global priority to support progress towards the SDGs. The Safe Childbirth Checklist (**Figures 1** and **2**) is a list of evidence-based practices derived from WHO guidelines [7–15] that target the major global causes of maternal deaths (haemorrhage, hypertensive disorders, infection, and obstructed labour), intrapartum-related stillbirths (inadequate intrapartum care) and neonatal deaths (intrapartum-related events, infection and complications of prematurity). Each checklist item is a critical action or practice that, if missed or left undone, can lead to severe harm for both the mother and or the newborn.

http://dx.doi.org/10.5772/intechopen.82616

BEFORE BIRTH

WHO Safe Childbirth Checklist

World Health Organization

1 On Admission

Does mother need referral? ☐ No ☐ Yes, organized	Check your facility's criteria
Partograph started? ☐ No, will start when ≥4cm ☐ Yes	Start plotting when cervix ≥4 cm, then cervix should dilate ≥1 cm/hr • Every 30 min: plot HR, contractions, fetal HR • Every 2 hrs: plot temperature • Every 4 hrs: plot BP
Does mother need to start: *Antibiotics?* ☐ No ☐ Yes, given	Ask for allergies before administration of any medication Give antibiotics to mother if any of: • Mother's temperature ≥38°C • History of foul-smelling vaginal discharge • Rupture of membranes >18 hrs
Magnesium sulfate and antihypertensive treatment? ☐ No ☐ Yes, magnesium sulfate given ☐ Yes, antihypertensive medication given	Give magnesium sulfate to mother if any of: • Diastolic BP ≥110 mmHg and 3+ proteinuria • Diastolic BP ≥90 mmHg, 2+ proteinuria, and any: severe headache, visual disturbance, epigastric pain Give antihypertensive medication to mother if systolic BP >160 mmHg • Goal: keep BP <150/100 mmHg
☐ **Confirm supplies are available to clean hands and wear gloves for each vaginal exam.**	
☐ **Encourage birth companion to be present at birth.**	
☐ **Confirm that mother or companion will call for help during labour if needed.**	Call for help if any of: • Bleeding • Severe abdominal pain • Severe headache or visual disturbance • Unable to urinate • Urge to push

This checklist is not intended to be comprehensive and should not replace the case notes or partograph. Additions and modifications to fit local practice are encouraged. For more information on recommended use of the checklist, please refer to the "WHO Safe Childbirth Checklist Implementation Guide" at: www.who.int/patientsafety.

WHO/HIS/SDS/2015.26

WHO Safe Childbirth Checklist

Completed by ____________________

BEFORE BIRTH

WHO Safe Childbirth Checklist

World Health Organization

2 Just Before Pushing (Or Before Caesarean)

Does mother need to start:

Antibiotics?

☐ No

☐ Yes, given

Ask for allergies before administration of any medication

Give antibiotics to mother if any of:

- Mother's temperature ≥38 °C
- History of foul-smelling vaginal discharge
- Rupture of membranes >18 hrs
- Caesarean section

Magnesium sulfate and antihypertensive treatment?

☐ No

☐ Yes, magnesium sulfate given

☐ Yes, antihypertensive medication given

Give magnesium sulfate to mother if any of:

- Diastolic BP ≥110 mmHg and 3+ proteinuria
- Diastolic BP ≥90 mmHg, 2+ proteinuria, and any: severe headache, visual disturbance, epigastric pain

Give antihypertensive medication to mother if systolic BP >160 mmHg

- Goal: keep BP <150/100 mmHg

Confirm essential supplies are at bedside and prepare for delivery:

For mother

☐ Gloves

☐ Alcohol-based handrub or soap and clean water

☐ Oxytocin 10 units in syringe

Prepare to care for mother immediately after birth:

Confirm single baby only (not multiple birth)

1. Give oxytocin within 1 minute after birth
2. Deliver placenta 1-3 minutes after birth
3. Massage uterus after placenta is delivered
4. Confirm uterus is contracted

For baby

☐ Clean towel

☐ Tie or cord clamp

☐ Sterile blade to cut cord

☐ Suction device

☐ Bag-and-mask

Prepare to care for baby immediately after birth:

1. Dry baby, keep warm
2. If not breathing, stimulate and clear airway
3. If still not breathing:
   - clamp and cut cord
   - clean airway if necessary
   - ventilate with bag-and-mask
   - shout for help

☐ **Assistant identified and ready to help at birth if needed.**

This checklist is not intended to be comprehensive and should not replace the case notes or partograph. Additions and modifications to fit local practice are encouraged. For more information on recommended use of the checklist, please refer to the "WHO Safe Childbirth Checklist Implementation Guide" at: www.who.int/patientsafety.

WHO Safe Childbirth Checklist

Completed by ____________________

AFTER BIRTH

WHO Safe Childbirth Checklist

World Health Organization

3 Soon After Birth (Within 1 Hour)

Is mother bleeding abnormally?
☐ No
☐ Yes, shout for help

If bleeding abnormally:
- Massage uterus
- Consider more uterotonic
- Start IV fluids and keep mother warm
- Treat cause: uterine atony, retained placenta/fragments, vaginal tear, uterine rupture

Does mother need to start:

Antibiotics?
☐ No
☐ Yes, given

Ask for allergies before administration of any medication
Give antibiotics to mother if placenta manually removed or if mother's temperature ≥38 °C and any of:
- Chills
- Foul-smelling vaginal discharge

If the mother has a third or fourth degree of perineal tear give antibiotics to prevent infection

Magnesium sulfate and antihypertensive treatment?
☐ No
☐ Yes, magnesium sulfate given
☐ Yes, antihypertensive medication given

Give magnesium sulfate to mother if any of:
- Diastolic BP ≥110 mmHg and 3+ proteinuria
- Diastolic BP ≥90 mmHg, 2+ proteinuria, and any: severe headache, visual disturbance, epigastric pain

Give antihypertensive medication to mother if systolic BP >160 mmHg
- Goal: keep BP <150/100 mmHg

Does baby need:

Referral?
☐ No
☐ Yes, organized

Check your facility's criteria.

Antibiotics?
☐ No
☐ Yes, given

Give baby antibiotics if antibiotics given to mother for treatment of maternal infection during childbirth or if baby has any of:
- Respiratory rate >60/min or <30/min
- Chest in-drawing, grunting, or convulsions
- Poor movement on stimulation
- Baby's temperature <35 °C (and not rising after warming) or baby's temperature ≥38 °C

Special care and monitoring?
☐ No
☐ Yes, organized

Arrange special care/monitoring for baby if any:
- More than 1 month early
- Birth weight <2500 grams
- Needs antibiotics
- Required resuscitation

☐ **Started breastfeeding and skin-to-skin contact (if mother and baby are well).**

☐ **Confirm mother / companion will call for help if danger signs present.**

Completed by ______________________

AFTER BIRTH

WHO Safe Childbirth Checklist

World Health Organization

4 Before Discharge

☐ **Confirm stay at facility for 24 hours after delivery.**

Does mother need to start antibiotics?

☐ No
☐ Yes, given and delay discharge

Ask for allergies before administration of any medication
Give antibiotics to mother if any of:
- Mother's temperature ≥38 °C
- Foul-smelling vaginal discharge

Is mother's blood pressure normal?

☐ No, treat and delay discharge
☐ Yes

Give magnesium sulfate to mother if any of:
- Diastolic BP ≥110 mmHg and 3+ proteinuria
- Diastolic BP ≥90 mmHg, 2+ proteinuria, and any: severe headache, visual disturbance, epigastric pain

Give antihypertensive medication to mother if systolic BP >160 mmHg
- Goal: keep BP <150/100 mmHg

Is mother bleeding abnormally?

☐ No
☐ Yes, treat and delay discharge

If pulse >110 beats per minute and blood pressure <90 mmHg
- Start IV and keep mother warm
- Treat cause (hypovolemic shock)

Does baby need to start antibiotics?

☐ No
☐ Yes, give antibiotics, delay discharge, give special care

Give antibiotics to baby if any of:
- Respiratory rate >60/min or <30/min
- Chest in-drawing, grunting, or convulsions
- Poor movement on stimulation
- Baby's temperature <35°C (and not rising after warming) or baby's temperature ≥38°C
- Stopped breastfeeding well
- Umbilicus redness extending to skin or draining pus

Is baby feeding well?

☐ No, establish good breastfeeding practices and delay discharge
☐ Yes

☐ **Discuss and offer family planning options to mother.**

☐ **Arrange follow-up and confirm mother / companion will seek help if danger signs appear after discharge.**

Danger Signs

***Mother** has any of:*
- Bleeding
- Severe abdominal pain
- Severe headache or visual disturbance
- Breathing difficulty
- Fever or chills
- Difficulty emptying bladder
- Epigastric pain

***Baby** has any of:*
- Fast/difficult breathing
- Fever
- Unusually cold
- Stops feeding well
- Less activity than normal
- Whole body becomes yellow

WHO Safe Childbirth Checklist

Completed by ____________________

Figure 1. The WHO Safe Childbirth Checklist.

http://dx.doi.org/10.5772/intechopen.82616

BEFORE BIRTH

WHO Safe Childbirth Checklist

World Health Organization

Name: Folder No:

1 On Admission

Does mother need referral? ☐ No ☐ Yes, organized	Check your facility's criteria
Partograph started? ☐ No, will start when ≥4cm ☐ Yes	Start plotting when cervix ≥4 cm, then cervix should dilate ≥1 cm/hr • Every 30 min: plot HR, contractions, fetal HR • Every 2 hrs: plot temperature • Every 4 hrs: plot BP
Does mother need to start: *Antibiotics?* ☐ No ☐ Yes, given	Ask for allergies before administration of any medication Give antibiotics to mother if any of: • Mother's temperature ≥38°C • History of foul-smelling vaginal discharge • Rupture of membranes >18 hrs
Magnesium sulfate and antihypertensive treatment? ☐ No ☐ Yes, magnesium sulfate given ☐ Yes, antihypertensive medication given	Give magnesium sulfate to mother if any of: • Diastolic BP ≥110 mmHg and 3+ proteinuria • Diastolic BP ≥90 mmHg, 2+ proteinuria, and any: severe headache, visual disturbance, epigastric pain Give antihypertensive medication to mother if systolic BP >160 mmHg • Goal: keep BP <150/100 mmHg
☐ **Confirm supplies are available to clean hands and wear gloves for each vaginal exam.**	
☐ **Encourage birth companion to be present at birth.**	
NA ☐ **Confirm that mother or companion will call for help during labour if needed.**	Call for help if any of: • Bleeding • Severe abdominal pain • Severe headache or visual disturbance • Unable to urinate • Urge to push

This checklist is not intended to be comprehensive and should not replace the case notes or partograph. Additions and modifications to fit local practice are encouraged. For more information on recommended use of the checklist, please refer to the "WHO Safe Childbirth Checklist Implementation Guide" at: www.who.int/patientsafety.

WHO/HIS/SDS/2015.26

WHO Safe Childbirth Checklist

Completed by ____________________

BEFORE BIRTH

WHO Safe Childbirth Checklist

World Health Organization

Name: Folder No:

2 Just Before Pushing (Or Before Caesarean)

Does mother need to start:

Antibiotics?

☐ No
☐ Yes, given

Ask for allergies before administration of any medication
Give antibiotics to mother if any of:

- Mother's temperature ≥38 °C
- History of foul-smelling vaginal discharge
- Rupture of membranes >18 hrs
- Caesarean section

Magnesium sulfate and antihypertensive treatment?

☐ No
☐ Yes, magnesium sulfate given
☐ Yes, antihypertensive medication given

Give magnesium sulfate to mother if any of:

- Diastolic BP ≥110 mmHg and 3+ proteinuria
- Diastolic BP ≥90 mmHg, 2+ proteinuria, and any: severe headache, visual disturbance, epigastric pain

Give antihypertensive medication to mother if systolic BP >160 mmHg

- Goal: keep BP <150/100 mmHg

Confirm essential supplies are at bedside and prepare for delivery:

For mother

☐ Gloves
☐ Alcohol-based handrub or soap and clean water
☐ Oxytocin 10 units in syringe

Prepare to care for mother immediately after birth:
Confirm single baby only (not multiple birth)

1. Give oxytocin within 1 minute after birth
2. Deliver placenta 1-3 minutes after birth
3. Massage uterus after placenta is delivered
4. Confirm uterus is contracted

For baby

☐ Clean towel
☐ Sterile blade to cut cord
☐ Suction device
☐ Bag-and-mask

Prepare to care for baby immediately after birth:

1. Dry baby, keep warm
2. If not breathing, stimulate and clear airway
3. If still not breathing:
   - clamp and cut cord
   - clean airway if necessary
   - ventilate with bag-and-mask
   - shout for help

☐ **Assistant identified and ready to help at birth if needed.**

This checklist is not intended to be comprehensive and should not replace the case notes or partograph. Additions and modifications to fit local practice are encouraged. For more information on recommended use of the checklist, please refer to the "WHO Safe Childbirth Checklist Implementation Guide" at: www.who.int/patientsafety.

WHO Safe Childbirth Checklist

Completed by ____________________

http://dx.doi.org/10.5772/intechopen.82616

AFTER BIRTH

WHO Safe Childbirth Checklist

World Health Organization

Name: Folder No:

3 Soon After Birth (Within 1 Hour)

Is mother bleeding abnormally?

☐ No

☐ Yes, shout for help

If bleeding abnormally:

- Massage uterus
- Consider more uterotonic
- Start IV and keep mother warm
- Treat cause: uterine atony, retained placenta/fragments, vaginal tear, uterine rupture

Does mother need to start:

Antibiotics?

☐ No

☐ Yes, given

Ask for allergies before administration of any medication

Give antibiotics to mother if placenta manually removed or if mother's temperature ≥38 °C and any of:

- Chills
- Foul-smelling vaginal discharge

If the mother has a third or fourth degree of perineal tear give antibiotics to prevent infection

Magnesium sulfate and antihypertensive treatment?

☐ No

☐ Yes, magnesium sulfate given

☐ Yes, antihypertensive medication given

Give magnesium sulfate to mother if any of:

- Diastolic BP ≥110 mmHg and 3+ proteinuria
- Diastolic BP ≥90 mmHg, 2+ proteinuria, and any: severe headache, visual disturbance, epigastric pain

Give antihypertensive medication to mother if systolic BP >160 mmHg

- Goal: keep BP <150/100 mmHg

Does baby need:

Referral?

☐ No

☐ Yes, given

Check your facility's criteria.

Antibiotics?

☐ No

☐ Yes, given

Give baby antibiotics if antibiotics given to mother for treatment of maternal infection during childbirth or if baby has any of:

- Respiratory rate >60/min or <30/min
- Chest in-drawing, grunting, or convulsions
- Poor movement on stimulation
- Baby's temperature <35 °C (and not rising after warming) or baby's temperature ≥38 °C

Special care and monitoring?

☐ No

☐ Yes, organized

Arrange special care/monitoring for baby if any:

- More than 1 month early
- Birth weight <2500 grams
- Needs antibiotics
- Required resuscitation

☐ **Started breastfeeding and skin-to-skin contact (if mother and baby are well).**

☐ **Confirm mother / companion will call for help if danger signs present.**

Completed by ______________

AFTER BIRTH

WHO Safe Childbirth Checklist

World Health Organization

Name: Folder No:

4 Before Discharge

☐ **Confirm stay at facility for 24 hours after delivery.**

Does mother need to start antibiotics? ☐ No ☐ Yes, given and delay discharge	Ask for allergies before administration of any medication Give antibiotics to mother if any of: • Mother's temperature ≥38 °C • Foul-smelling vaginal discharge
Is mother's blood pressure normal? ☐ No, treat and delay discharge ☐ Yes	Give magnesium sulfate to mother if any of: • Diastolic BP ≥110 mmHg and 3+ proteinuria • Diastolic BP ≥90 mmHg, 2+ proteinuria, and any: severe headache, visual disturbance, epigastric pain Give antihypertensive medication to mother if systolic BP >160 mmHg • Goal: keep BP <150/100 mmHg
Is mother bleeding abnormally? ☐ No ☐ Yes, treat and delay discharge	If pulse >110 beats per minute and blood pressure <90 mmHg • Start IV and keep mother warm • Treat cause (hypovolemic shock)
Does baby need to start antibiotics? ☐ No ☐ Yes, give antibiotics, delay discharge, give special care	Give antibiotics to baby if any of: • Respiratory rate >60/min or <30/min • Chest in-drawing, grunting, or convulsions • Poor movement on stimulation • Baby's temperature <35°C (and not rising after warming) or baby's temperature ≥38°C • Stopped breastfeeding well • Umbilicus redness extending to skin or draining pus

Is baby feeding well?

☐ No, establish good breastfeeding practices and delay discharge
☐ Yes

☐ **Discuss and offer family planning options to mother.**

☐ **Arrange follow-up and confirm mother / companion will seek help if danger signs appear after discharge.**

Danger Signs

Mother *has any of:*

- Bleeding
- Severe abdominal pain
- Severe headache or visual disturbance
- Breathing difficulty
- Fever or chills
- Difficulty emptying bladder
- Epigastric pain

Baby *has any of:*

- Fast/difficult breathing
- Fever
- Unusually cold
- Stops feeding well
- Less activity than normal
- Whole body becomes yellow

WHO Safe Childbirth Checklist Completed by ____________

Figure 2. The WHO Safe Childbirth Checklist adapted for UPTH ©Rosemary Ogu.

http://dx.doi.org/10.5772/intechopen.82616

2. Methodology

This chapter utilises experiences gained in Cameroon, Ghana, Nigeria and Zambia during the Pfizer Independent Grant for Learning and Change supported Medical Women's Association of Nigeria Improving Maternal Health in sub-Saharan Africa project to describe how the checklist can be used to deliver lifesaving midwifery care and enhance maternal health. This chapter also outlines the 'how to use the checklist' as elucidated in the WHO implementation guide in this chapter [4].

3. How to use the Checklist

This segment describes how to use the checklist to deliver life-saving birth practices. Tips on how to effectively use the checklist as a quality improvement tool, advocating and getting supplies for use in maternity units are included.

3.1. Pause points

The checklist is envisioned to be used at four points in time; these points are called 'pause points'. At each pause point, a set of essential practices; also known as the 'checklist items' should be completed. Each checklist item should be marked with a pen when that item is completed. The healthcare worker who is caring for the woman and baby at the time a pause point occurs should be responsible for completing the checklist then. Labour ward staff in Port Harcourt Nigeria found the checklist facilitated best practices and improved patient satisfaction with care [16].

Checklist users may be nurses, midwives, physicians, or other clinicians; as seen in Cameroon, Ghana and Nigeria. In Lusaka- Zambia, none of the sampled institutions were using the checklist. The recommended approach for using the checklist is for healthcare workers to first conduct their normal practice and then use the checklist to verify that the checklist items have been correctly performed. One checklist should be used for every mother and her baby; in Port Harcourt; the checklist was modified to include the mother's name and folder number (**Figure 2**).

There are four pause points. Pause points are therefore the specific point in time when staff are asked to temporarily stop whatever else they are doing and verify or check that essential clinical practices have been completed [4]. Pause points thus happen at critical moments in care when complications can be averted, or adequately treated; or when it is expedient for healthcare workers to check the woman and baby. The four pause points are:

1. at the time of admission;

2. just before the woman starts pushing (or before caesarean section);

3. within 1 h after birth; and

4. before discharge from the facility.

These pause points may not all occur in the same room. For instance, at the University of Port Harcourt Teaching Hospital Obstetric Unit in Nigeria and the Yaounde Gynaeco-Obstetric and Paediatric Hospital, Yaounde, Cameroon; pause point 1 takes place at the admission desk, pause point 2 occurs in the labour room, pause point 3 in the postpartum bay, and pause point 4 occurs in the postpartum ward. In other facilities that are small, or those implementing the recent recommendation that women should labour and deliver in the same room and on the same bed, all pause points will occur in a single area. If the pause points occur in separate areas, it is vital that the checklist accompany the woman and baby when they are moved from one area to the other. In our experiences, this is achieved by keeping the checklist with the woman's chart or inside her medical record folder.

3.2. Checklist items

The 'checklist items' are the set of evidence-based obstetric practices that should be carried out. They specifically address the major global causes of maternal and newborn deaths and comprise a core set of evidence-based practices that have been proven to reduce and prevent maternal and newborn harm. These practices are to be carried out at every birth. Supplemental information is available in the checklist for many items in order to improve care. This information is located adjacent to the checklist item it describes. For instance, the supplemental information for checklist items relating to medications describes the indications for antibiotic use. Dosages and treatment courses for all medications should be aligned with WHO or local guidelines. Every effort should be made to have supplies and consumables available for use when needed; otherwise, the indication will be present, but the health caregiver cannot implement the needed evidence base practice because the necessary supplies are unavailable. Our experiences show that in all instances, advocacy is necessary for improved supplies of equipment, tools, and consumables. Refresher courses periodically for health workers are also necessary to update and refresh knowledge.

After repeated use of the checklist, users may come to memorise the supplemental information. In these situations, users should still run the checklist by reviewing and marking each checklist item to be sure that all essential practices are conducted.

Each item on the Safe Childbirth Checklist is described in detail below.

3.2.1. Pause point 1: on admission

At the time of admission; evaluation of the mother is essential to review her general status, discover and manage complications that she may already have. An evaluation also confirms if referral to another facility is indicated. At this pause point, the woman and her companion are counselled for labour and delivery, educated about the danger signs and what to do thereafter.

3.2.1.1. Does mother need referral?

This checklist item ensures that mothers with indications for referral are promptly referred. Presentation in extremis is one reason why women die in health facilities. This must be avoided at all times. The WHO Checklist implementation guide [4] advises the skilled birth attendant confirm whether the mother needs a referral to another facility by reviewing the facility's criteria for a referral. If indicated, the guide [4] further advises the healthcare worker to take immediate action to organise a safe transfer.

The healthcare worker should inform the mother and birth companion about the need for the referral so they can act fast. Informing healthcare workers at the facility to which the mother is being referred enable the receiving facility to prepare and in a position to deliver care as soon as the mother arrives. This is imperative to save lives and minimise morbidity and mortality. A list of indications for referral in the admission area helps healthcare workers to quickly identify mothers that should be referred. Ensuring communication tools/means of transportation are available is essential in reducing maternal morbidity and mortality as experiences show that after referral; mothers in low resource settings may find it difficult to go to the referred facility due to financial constraints.

3.2.1.2. Partograph started?

The partograph is a tool that graphically represents the events in labour and thus assesses the progress of labour. The partographs alert and action lines enable birth attendants to recognise and take action to prevent and manage prolonged and obstructed labour. The use of the partograph prevents prolonged labour, reduces operative intervention, and improves neonatal outcomes [7]. The skilled birth attendant should fill out a partogram first page for every patient who comes on admission in the labour ward and start the partograph when active labour is established or when a mother's cervical dilation is 4 cm or more. Every 30 min, the mother's heart rate, number of contractions in 10 min, and the foetal heart rate should be checked and charted on the partograph. The mother's temperature should be checked every 2 h and plotted while her mother's blood pressure is checked and plotted every 4 h. If at the time of admission, the mother is not in active labour, then the partograph is attached to her chart or medical record folder. The partograph is then started when her cervical dilatation reaches 4 cm. Refresher courses on the use of partograph should be organised periodically for obstetric unit staff to enhance the use of the partograph in adequately monitoring labour.

3.2.1.3. Does mother need to start antibiotics?

Antibiotics prevent and treat bacterial infections. Antibiotics should ideally be stocked in the labour ward and administered as soon as indicated to improve outcomes. Antibiotic treatment prevents infection-related complications in the mother, the foetus, and in the newborn. The skilled birth attendant should confirm whether the mother needs antibiotics at the time of admission and if indicated; for example, if the mother has a temperature of or greater than 38°C, rupture of the membranes greater than 18 h or foul-smelling vaginal discharge; the antibiotics should be immediately administered. In Cameroon, use of the checklist in about 1000 deliveries revealed that infections complications are less when the checklist is in use compared to when the checklist is not in use.

3.2.1.4. Does mother need to start magnesium sulphate?

Magnesium sulphate is the gold standard for the prevention of Eclampsia. Pre-eclampsia is a severe form of hypertension or very high blood pressure in pregnancy (≥160/110 mmHg) with its associated complications of abruptio, eclampsia and stroke for the mother, and intrauterine foetal death for the baby. Prophylactic treatment of pre-eclampsia with magnesium sulphate and antihypertensive treatment prevents these complications. At this pause point at the time of admission, the Skilled birth attendant should confirm from the blood pressure reading and presence of proteinuria on urinalysis whether the mother needs magnesium sulphate and antihypertensive treatment. If yes, i.e. the mother has diastolic blood pressure equal to or greater than 110 mmHg with proteinuria of 3+, or if her diastolic blood pressure is equal to or greater than 90 mmHg with proteinuria of 2+ and any signs of pre-eclampsia (epigastric pain, severe headache or visual disturbance), the magnesium sulphate and antihypertensive agent should be urgently administered. Magnesium sulphate should continue for 24 h after childbirth or after the last convulsion. High blood pressure should be confirmed by the measurement of blood pressure on more than one occasion. If the mothers systolic blood pressure is equal to or greater than 160 mmHg, antihypertensives should be administered to lower and maintain blood pressure to just below 150/100 mmHg. If magnesium sulphate can only be administered after the patient has procured it, the patient financial constraints imply indicated magnesium sulphate is not administered when needed and foetomaternal outcomes remain poor similar to the experiences in India [17].

3.2.1.5. *Does mother need to start antiretrovirals?*

Transmission of HIV from positive mothers to their babies can occur during childbirth. Antiretroviral treatment (ART) reduce this risk. The skilled birth attendant should confirm whether the mother needs antiretrovirals at the time of admission and, if indicated, the antiretrovirals should be immediately administered. If the mother's HIV status is unknown, then an HIV test should done. If a pregnant woman tests HIV-positive, then antiretroviral drugs should be administered and continued throughout labour, delivery, breastfeeding, and thereafter.

3.2.1.6. *Confirm supplies are available near bedside to clean hands and wear gloves for each vaginal exam*

This checklist item is so very necessary because healthcare workers with unclean hands can spread infections to mothers and babies. Practicing good hand hygiene prevents these infections. Puerperal sepsis is a major global cause of morbidity and mortality for mothers and babies. Healthcare workers should thus always thoroughly wash their hands with soap and clean water before and after they make contact with clients. If water is unavailable, as can happen in low resource setting; an alcohol-based hand rub should be used. Advocacy for hygiene supplies (i.e. soap, clean running water, or alcohol-based hand rub, clean gloves) must be included in the engagement with heads of facilities. Availability at all times promotes healthcare workers adherence to good hand hygiene practices. Correct techniques for hand hygiene should be practiced. This is so very important to improve outcomes. Availability of the checklist and its use in a setting of a dearth of clean water and consumables implies that foetomaternal outcomes will remain poor.

3.2.1.7. *Encourage birth companion to be present at birth*

Available evidence show that birth companions can help to improve health outcomes by providing support to the mother during the childbirth process. Birth companions can help to recognise danger signs, and thus alert the healthcare worker. A birth companion could be a family member, husband, partner, friend, community health worker, or facility staff. The checklist implementation guide advocates that skilled birth attendant should encourage the presence of a birth companion during labour, birth, and the postpartum and postnatal periods [4]. The implementation guide [4] further encourages that a birth companion is present at the time of admission; and if a birth companion is not present at the time of admission, then the mother should be encouraged to identify one; the birth companion should be counselled on danger signs and encouraged to stay through the entire childbirth process.

3.2.1.8. Confirm that mother or companion will call for help during labour if needed

At the time of admission; the checklist encourages the healthcare worker to confirm that the parturient or birth companion will call for help if needed, if she feels like pushing and if any danger signs develop during labour: bleeding, severe abdominal pain, severe headache or visual disturbance, or inability to urinate. This is imperative as these danger signs portend complications which: are unpredictable, may happen at any time during childbirth and become more challenging to manage the longer they go undetected and untreated. It is thus crucial that healthcare workers detect and manage complications early. 'Danger signs' are signs and symptoms that reveal a complication may be developing or is already present. Many times, healthcare workers will recognise danger signs directly. However, due to the busy nature of the labour ward, the health worker is preoccupied at the instance a danger sign develops in a mother or baby. Thus, it is essential the parturient and her birth companion are vigilant and alert the healthcare workers. Findings reveal that many women are unaware of the danger signs in labour [18–20]. Mothers and birth companions should therefore be educated to recognise danger signs and to alert a healthcare worker immediately.

3.2.2. Pause point 2: just before pushing (or before caesarean)

After admission, the foetomaternal vital signs are monitored routinely. A deliberate check should be taken at pause point 2 which is the next pause point after admission; just before pushing or before a caesarean section. This allows the detection of complications that can occur during labour and enables the treatment. This pause point helps to prepare for the routine events and possible crisis situations that can occur.

3.2.2.1. Does mother need to start antibiotics?

As stated above, antibiotics help to prevent and treat infections. The Skilled birth attendant should confirm whether the mother needs antibiotics at the time that pushing starts or just before caesarean and, if indicated, the antibiotics should immediately be administered. The indications for antibiotics are a maternal temperature of 38°C or higher, membranes rupture greater than 18 h or foul-smelling vaginal discharge. All women undergoing caesarean delivery should receive antibiotics before skin incision.

3.2.2.2. Does mother need to start magnesium sulphate and antihypertensive treatment?

This question must be asked at this pause point as hypertensive disorders of pregnancy is a global cause of maternal mortality and morbidity. Between the time of admission and just before pushing; pre-eclampsia can arise. Prophylactic treatment with magnesium sulphate and antihypertensive medicines will help prevent maternal and perinatal mortality and morbidity. The Skilled birth attendant should confirm whether the mother needs magnesium sulphate and antihypertensive treatment at the time that the second stage starts, and if indicated, magnesium sulphate should be administered immediately and blood pressure lowered with antihypertensives. Magnesium sulphate should continue for 24 h after childbirth or 24 h after the last convulsion.

3.2.2.3. Confirm essential supplies are at the bedside and prepare for delivery

The time of highest risk for complications in the mother and her newborn is the moment of birth and the first few minutes after birth. Availability of functioning equipment and supplies is key to preventing maternal and neonatal mortality and morbidity at this time. Crisis situations can evolve quickly, and healthcare workers will not have enough time to prepare once in a crisis situation. Therefore, preparations must be made beforehand for both routine care and potential crisis situations at every birth. Specifically, healthcare workers must prepare essential supplies and also prepare themselves to take essential actions. Advocacy to hospital managers should be undertaken [21], and innovation for supplies availability periodically carried out. The essential supplies must always be available, functioning and ready to use before the birth occurs.

Confirm that a ready packed delivery tray is available by the bedside. The tray should contain the following essential supplies: Gloves; Episiotomy and cord scissors, cord clamp, Syringe and Oxytocin, a clean towel to dry the baby immediately after birth, a suction device, and bag-and-mask. Confirm actions to prevent post-partum bleeding: administer 10 IU of oxytocin intramuscularly to the mother within 1 min of delivery; clamp and cut the cord before ensuring complete delivery of the placenta by controlled cord traction; massage the uterus immediately after the delivery of the placenta. These components of the active management of the third stage of labour help the uterus to contract and prevents bleeding.

The use of clean towels to dry the baby helps retain warmth while the suction device clears secretions from the baby's mouth and nose. These simple devices and actions help keep the baby alive.

As described in the WHO checklist implementation guide [4]; at pause point 2, the skilled birth attendant should review the steps involved in care for the baby immediately after birth to ensure a successful transition to extrauterine life.

3.2.2.4. Assistant identified and ready to help at birth if needed

Recall in pause point 1, the moment of childbirth and the first few minutes after are the time of highest risk for complications in the mother, and the baby. If a crisis occurs, the presence of an available assistant helps. They can assist in assessing the mother or baby, starting IV fluids, administering medications, organising referrals and calling for additional help.

3.2.2.5. Is the mother bleeding abnormally?

Obstetric haemorrhage is a major cause of maternal morbidity and mortality that must be detected and treated as soon as possible. It occurs because of uterine rupture, abruptio placenta, and placenta praevia. At this pause point; also assess the pulse of the mother: the first signs of hypovolemic shock is a rising pulse rate. The skilled birth attendant should thus assess the mother for abnormal bleeding at this pause point just before pushing and if the mother is bleeding abnormally: call for help, expedite delivery and treat the specific cause of the abnormal bleeding.

3.2.3. Pause point 3: soon after birth (within 1 h)

At this pause point; complications that can occur soon after delivery can be detected and treated promptly if the mother and baby are reviewed soon after birth (within 1 h). This point also provides opportunity to educate the mother (and her companion) about danger signs for which she should call for help.

3.2.3.1. Is the mother bleeding abnormally?

Postpartum haemorrhage is a dreaded cause of morbidity and mortality. It is a major complication that must be detected and treated early if mortality and morbidity are to be averted. Postpartum bleeding can occur because of uterine atony, retained placenta or placental fragments, a vaginal tear, a cervical tear, or uterine rupture. Abnormal bleeding is defined as blood loss of 500 ml or any blood loss in which the mother's condition deteriorates. Thus, action must be taken at lower blood loss if a mother is severely anaemic. The skilled birth attendant should assess the mother for abnormal bleeding soon after birth (within 1 h) and if the mother is bleeding abnormally: massage the uterus, administer more uterotonic such as oxytocin, misoprostol, IV fluids, and treat the specific cause of the abnormal bleeding.

3.2.3.2. Does mother need to start antibiotics?

The Skilled birth attendant should confirm whether the mother needs antibiotics soon after birth (within 1 h) and, if indicated; for instance, if the mother's placenta was removed manually, she sustained a third or fourth degree perineal tear, or she has a temperature of 38°C or higher and chills, or foul-smelling vaginal discharge; the antibiotics should be administered immediately.

3.2.3.3. Does mother need to start magnesium sulphate and antihypertensive treatment?

A systolic blood pressure of more than 160 mmHg requires antihypertensive medications to lower and prevent eclampsia. Hypertensive disorders in pregnancy after delivery of the baby is a challenge; over 30% of eclamptic fits occur after childbirth. Thus, the Skilled birth attendant should confirm at this pause point whether the mother needs magnesium sulphate and antihypertensive treatment and, if indicated, the magnesium sulphate should be administered immediately. Remember to continue the magnesium sulphate for 24 or until 24 h after the last fit in mothers who had eclampsia.

3.2.3.4. Does baby need referral?

At this pause point after delivery, babies with complications should be reviewed and if necessary; referred to another facility. The Skilled birth attendant should thus confirm if baby needs referral within 1 h of delivery and expedite the process of a safe transfer. Pasting a list of referral criteria in the postnatal area can serve as a useful reminder for healthcare workers and enable them to quickly identify babies who should be referred. The reason for referral should be made known to the mother and to healthcare workers at the receiving facility. Arrangements for the fastest means of transportation should be planned ahead of time.

3.2.3.5. Does baby need antibiotics?

Within 1 h after childbirth, the Skilled birth attendant should confirm whether the baby needs antibiotics and, if indicated, the antibiotics should be administered immediately to prevent infection related complications. Indications for antibiotics in newborns include maternal antibiotics administration, neonatal temperature <35°C or ≥38°C, neonatal respiratory rate >60 per minute or <30 per minute, chest indrawing, grunting, or convulsions; or poor movement on stimulation.

3.2.3.6. Does baby need special care or monitoring?

This checklist item is necessary because some babies may have risk factors that do not meet the criteria for referral, but for which special care or monitoring is yet required. Thus to be safe, such babies must receive special care. The indications are listed on the checklist and include baby is born more than 1 month early, has a low birthweight <2500 g, needs antibiotics or required resuscitation to help cry or breathe at birth.

3.2.3.7. Start breastfeeding and skin-to-skin contact (if mother and baby are well)

The Skilled birth attendant should confirm that breastfeeding and skin-to-skin contact have been started soon after birth (within 1 h). This is a practice that is free; every effort should be made to ensure it is carried out. Early breastfeeding is best. Evidence shows that early breastfeeding within 1 h of birth stimulate uterine contraction through oxytocin release, prevent postpartum haemorrhage and helps the baby to establish good bonding with the mother. Similarly, skin-to-skin contact of the baby with the mother is the best method for keeping the baby warm and helps to promote bonding between the baby and the mother. Complications can quickly occur if a baby's core temperature falls below the normal range. Skin-to-skin contact is done by placing the baby's skin against the mother's skin, and a clean sheet or blanket wrapped around them.

3.2.3.8. Confirm mother/companion will call for help if danger signs present

This checklist item reiterates the importance of danger sign awareness in newborns/mothers. Thus mothers (and birth companions) should be educated to recognise danger signs and to alert a healthcare worker immediately they discover a danger sign such as fast breathing or difficulty breathing, fever, unusually cold, not feeding well, less activity than normal, or the whole body becomes yellow. Also danger signs in mothers such as severe headache or visual disturbance, bleeding, severe abdominal pain, difficulty breathing, chills or fever or difficulty emptying her bladder.

3.2.4. Pause point 4: before discharge

The condition of mother and baby can deteriorate fast; the healthcare worker should check the mother and baby for signs or symptoms such as breathlessness, jaundice, poor suck, feeling tired or too weak to get out of bed. The checklist items at this pause point ensure that the mother and baby are reviewed and evaluated before discharge, and adjudged mother and baby are healthy before discharge. This point also reminds the healthcare worker to arrange for follow-up care, ensure family planning options have been discussed and offered, and further educate the mother (and her companion) about possible danger signs after discharge from facility.

3.2.4.1. *Confirm stay at facility for 24 h after delivery*

This checklist item is to ensure mothers and newborns are at a place where care can be given should any complication arise. Evidence shows that half of all maternal deaths and 40% of neonatal deaths occur during the first 24 h after childbirth. The WHO, therefore, recommends that the mother and her newborn be observed in the health facility for at least 24 h after childbirth (before discharge). This is the ideal. However, our experiences reveal that lack of bed space in postnatal wards implies well mothers are discharged home early before 24 h after delivery.

3.2.4.2. *Does mother need to start antibiotics?*

This checklist item is at this pause point because puerperal sepsis is a major cause of maternal mortality and morbidity. The Healthcare worker should therefore confirm if the mother needs antibiotics before discharge and, if indicated, the discharge should be delayed while the antibiotics should be administered immediately. Indications for antibiotics include a maternal temperature of 38°C or higher, chills or foul-smelling vaginal discharge. Mastitis or infection of a caesarean section wound are troublesome conditions which may not be present at the time of discharge; thus women should be educated and counselled to report at the facility if these problems occur after discharge.

3.2.4.3. *Is mother's blood pressure normal?*

Before discharge of the mother, the Healthcare worker should check to ensure that the blood pressure is normal as preeclampsia can arise after childbirth and one-third of all the eclamptic seizures appear during the postpartum period. Also, following postpartum haemorrhage, normal blood pressure is a sign of stable condition. Thus all mothers must have a blood pressure check at the time of discharge.

3.2.4.4. *Is mother bleeding abnormally?*

The healthcare worker should ascertain whether the mother's bleeding is controlled before discharge and whether the pulse is normal. Examine the mother's abdomen to be sure the uterus is contracted and check blood loss from the vagina. If the mother's pulse rate is high, it may indicate that she is still bleeding, the mother should be treated, and not discharged. No mother with a high pulse rate or bleeding should be discharged.

3.2.4.5. *Does baby need to start antibiotics?*

Bacterial infections are a major cause of death in newborn babies. The healthcare worker should confirm whether the baby needs antibiotics before discharge and, if indicated, antibiotics should be administered immediately, the discharge should be delayed and special care or monitoring should be given. Indications for antibiotics in newborns include: maternal antibiotics administration, neonatal temperature <35°C or ≥38°C, neonatal respiratory rate >60 per minute or <30 per minute; chest indrawing, grunting, or convulsions; or poor movement on stimulation, umbilicus redness extending to skin or draining pus; poor movement on stimulation; or has stopped breastfeeding well. It is imperative that babies with infection or risk factors for infection are treated immediately to prevent infection-related complications.

3.2.4.6. Is baby feeding well?

This checklist item prompts the healthcare worker to confirm before the mother and baby are discharged from the birth facility; that adequate breastfeeding has been established. In a baby; the signs of feeding well are active breastfeeding every 1–3 h with urination and bowel motions. If the newborn is not feeding well, the healthcare worker should delay discharge and assist the mother in establishing good feeding.

3.2.4.7. Discuss and offer family planning options to mother

This checklist item ensures the healthcare worker will remember to offer family planning options to the mother before her discharge. Recall that after a live birth, the recommended interval before attempting the next pregnancy is around 2 years. Family planning helps to prevent unwanted pregnancies and safeguards the mother. The healthcare worker should confirm that family planning options have been discussed with and offered to the mother before discharge. Family planning options include intrauterine devices, implantable rods, long-acting injectable progesterone (Depo-Provera), oral contraceptives, tubal ligation and condoms. Intra-uterine devices can be inserted immediately after childbirth, during or after the 6 weeks postpartum visit. Implantable devices (Implanon, Jadelle) can be inserted immediately after childbirth or after the puerperium. Breastfeeding mothers are generally advised not use combined hormonal contraceptives before 6 months postpartum. Health care workers using Checklist should also take the opportunity before discharge of the mother to discuss optimal birth spacing and schedule a tubal ligation procedure for mothers who wish.

3.2.4.8. Arrange follow-up and confirm mother/companion will seek help if danger signs appear after discharge

This checklist item ensures the healthcare worker arranges for routine follow-up for both the mother and baby. This must be arranged for before the mother-baby pair are discharged from the hospital. A healthy mother and baby at the time of discharge may develop complications after they have returned home. Mothers (and birth companions) should thus be educated to recognise danger signs themselves so care can be requested promptly: The danger signs are:

bleeding, severe abdominal pain, severe headache or visual disturbance, difficulty breathing, fever or chills, difficulty emptying bladder, or epigastric pain in the mother while in the baby; fast breathing or difficulty breathing, unusually cold, fever, stopping to feed well, less activity than normal, or whole body becoming yellow.

4. Discussion

Using the WHO Safe Childbirth Checklist serves as a powerful reminder of all that needs to be done during the critical period of childbirth. It also highlights the deficiencies in maternity service delivery: the dearth of manpower resources; the absence of antibiotics, anticonvulsants, antihypertensives and oxytocics; the lack of necessary supplies and commodities such as gloves, antiseptic lotions, clean towels, swabs, syringes; the unavailability of water supply and electricity; and the sociocultural determinants that make women present to health facilities in extremis.

Gaining, and sourcing for dedicated healthcare workers to champion the cause of the childbirth checklist revealed the dearth of human resources for health. Advocacy and dedication are vital at this point to introduce the checklist for use in maternity settings. Making the checklist available at the point of care is the next hurdle. Simple paper and ink may not be available, but a satisfactory buy-in by the facility managers ensure the checklist is printed and available at the necessary points. The need to ensure the available number of healthcare workers using the childbirth checklist can satisfactorily carry out the evidence base practices lead to training and workforce skills enhancement. This strengthened the services provided at the facilities.

On admission, using the checklist immediately exposes the absence of facility guidelines and criteria on whom to refer; thus effectively using the checklist strengthens the facility to provide guidelines and facility criteria for referral. At the same time; risk factors for poor maternal/perinatal outcomes such as prolonged drainage of liquor, fever, high blood pressure and proteinuria are easily detected because the healthcare worker must check these in order to tick the checklist. Same for the use of partograph; to tick the checklist, the healthcare worker has to open and use the partograph. To tick and confirm that mother or companion will call for help during labour if needed, the healthcare worker has to first counsel and educate the mother and her companion on the danger signs in pregnancy; these are usually not routinely done. Users of the checklist in Port Harcourt, Nigeria, and Yaounde, Cameroon, confirmed that the checklist helped them to counsel patients better.

At the various pause points: just before pushing (or before caesarean), soon after birth, or just before discharge; using the checklist helps to prepare for a safe, positive childbirth experience thus averting morbidity and mortality. Although the childbirth checklist does not introduce any new interventions for safe childbirth; the use reveals when the evidence-based interventions for safe childbirth were not being implemented; partographs not being used, handwashing not being carried out, anticonvulsants not being administered for women with severe preeclampsia, active management of the third stage of labour not being rigorously followed; antibiotics not administered religiously before caesarean sections and skin contact for babies following deliveries not being implemented. These were the experiences we had as users of the checklist in sub-Saharan Africa. All in all; the evidence-based practices for safe childbirth were not being religiously implemented across the obstetric units mostly because of financial constraints and a dearth of human resources. The workforce skills upgrade was the first to improve; however skills alone is not enough to change outcomes; it improved satisfaction with work done; with care received, but with overall morbidity and mortality reduction, the change is not readily visible.

To enable visible change in maternal and perinatal morbidity and mortality outcomes, users of the checklist must in addition to workforce skills training and coaching, advocate for supplies and commodities availability. When antibiotics, anticonvulsants, oxytocics, antiseptics, water, electricity and safe childbirth checklist are available, effective delivery of services, counselling and respectful maternity care leads to improved maternal and perinatal outcomes.

5. Conclusion

Using the Safe Childbirth Checklist ensures the delivery of essential maternal and perinatal midwifery care practices. The Safe Childbirth Checklist addresses the major causes of maternal deaths, intrapartum-related stillbirths, and neonatal deaths and enables the caregiver to anticipate and avert complications. It also enables the caregiver to acknowledge the limitations/gaps in the currently available health service delivery unit and advocate for supplies and equipment. It has the potential to facilitate compliance with best practices for the delivery of evidence-based better birth. Complications from obstetric haemorrhage, infection, obstructed labour, hypertensive disorders, inadequate intrapartum care, birth asphyxia, infection, and complications related to prematurity can be minimised if the tenets of the checklist are followed. Its use in obstetric units is therefore advocated.

Acknowledgements

The authors thank Pfizer for the Pfizer Independent Grant for Learning and Change (Pfizer IGLC) ID Number 33584051; the World Health Organisation Patient Safety and Quality Improvement Unit, Geneva, Switzerland; Dr Clarissa Fabre & Dr Shelley Ross of Medical Women International Association for their support.

Conflict of interest

The authors declare no conflict of interest.

Author details

Julius Dohbit[1], Vetty Agala[2,3], Pamela Chinwa-Banda[4], Betty Anane-Fenin[5], Omosivie Maduka[3,6], Ufuoma Edewor[3], Ibimonye Porbeni[3], Fru Angwafo[1] and Rosemary Ogu[3,7]*

*Address all correspondence to: rosemary.ogu@uniport.edu.ng

1 The Yaounde Gynaeco-Obstetric and Paediatric Hospital, The University of Yaounde I, Yaounde, Cameroon

2 Department of Community Medicine, University of Port Harcourt Teaching Hospital, Port Harcourt, Nigeria

3 Medical Women's Association of Nigeria, Rivers State Branch, Port Harcourt, Nigeria

4 Ministry of General Education, Lusaka, Zambia

5 Department of Obstetrics and Gynaecology, Cape Coast Teaching Hospital, Cape Coast, Ghana

6 Department of Preventive and Social Medicine, University of Port Harcourt, Port Harcourt, Nigeria

7 Department of Obstetrics and Gynaecology, University of Port Harcourt, Port Harcourt, Nigeria

References

[1] WHO. WHO Maternal Mortality Factsheet 2015. Available from: http://www.who.int/mediacentre/factsheets/fs348/en/ [Cited: July 29, 2018]

[2] Ogu RN, Agholor KN, Okonofua FE. Engendering the attainment of the SDG-3 in Africa: Overcoming the socio-cultural factors contributing to maternal mortality. African Journal of Reproductive Health. 2016;**20**(3):62-74

[3] Ogu RN, Ntoimo LF, Okonofua FE. Perceptions of women on workloads in health facilities and its effect on maternal health care: A multi-site qualitative study in Nigeria. Midwifery. 2017;**55**(12):1-6

[4] WHO. WHO Safe Childbirth Checklist Implementation Guide: Improving the Quality of Facility-Based Delivery for Mothers and Newborns [Internet]. 2015. Available from: http://www.who.int/patientsafety/implementation/checklists/childbirth-checklist_implementation-guide/en/ [Cited: July 26, 2018]

[5] Gawande A. The Checklist Manifesto: How to Get Things Right. New York: Metropolitan Books; 2010

[6] Barnes C, Berry W, Edmondson L, et al. Safe Surgery Checklist Implementation Guide. Boston, MA: Ariadne Labs; 2015. Available from: www.SafeSurgery2015.org

[7] World Health Organisation. World Health Organization partograph in management of labour. Lancet. 1994;**343**:1399-1404. DOI: https://doi.org/10.1016/S0140-6736(94)92528-3

[8] WHO, United Nations Population Fund, UNICEF. Pregnancy, Childbirth, Postpartum and Newborn Care: A Guide for Essential Practice. Geneva: World Health Organization; 2015. ISBN: 9789241549356

[9] World Health Organisation. WHO Recommendations for Prevention and Treatment of Pre-eclampsia and Eclampsia. Geneva: World Health Organization; 2011. ISBN: 978924 1548335

[10] World Health Organisation. WHO Guidelines on Basic Newborn Resuscitation. Geneva: World Health Organization; 2012. ISBN: 9789241503693

[11] World Health Organisation. WHO Recommendations on Postnatal Care of the Mother and Newborn: Highlights from the World Health Organization 2013 Guidelines. Geneva: World Health Organization; 2015. ISBN: 9789241506649

[12] World Health Organisation. Consolidated Guidelines on the Use of Antiretroviral Drugs for Treating and Preventing HIV Infection. Geneva: The World Health Organization; 2016. ISBN: 9789241549684

[13] World Health Organisation. Guidelines for the Treatment of Malaria. 3rd ed. Geneva: World Health Organization; 2015. ISBN: 9789241549127

[14] WHO Recommendations on Interventions to Improve Preterm Birth Outcomes. France: World Health Organization; 2015. ISBN: 9789241508988

[15] WHO. Medical Eligibility Criteria for Contraceptive Use. 2015. Available from: http://apps.who.int/iris/bitstream/10665/181468/1/9789241549158_eng.pdf

[16] Ogu R, Tobin-West C, Orazulike N, John O, Maduka O, Inimgba N, et al. Improving maternal health: Implementing the WHO Safe Childbirth Checklist facilitates compliance with best practices. British Journal of Obstetrics and Gynaecology. 2017;**124**:26-35. DOI: 10.1111/1471-0528.8_14571

[17] Semrau KEA, Hirschhorn LR, Marx Delaney M, Singh VP, Saurastri R, Sharma N, et al. Outcomes of a coaching-based WHO Safe Childbirth Checklist Program in India. The New England Journal of Medicine. 2017;**377**(24):2313-2324

[18] Ogu RN, Orazulike NC. Reducing maternal mortality: Awareness of danger signs in pregnancy. Asian Journal of Medicine and Health. 2017;**6**(1):1-8

[19] Bogale D, Markos D. Knowledge of obstetric danger signs among child bearing age women in Goba district, Ethiopia: A cross-sectional study. BMC Pregnancy and Childbirth. 2015;**15**:77

[20] Bililign N, Mulatu T. Knowledge of obstetric danger signs and associated factors among reproductive age women in Raya Kobo district of Ethiopia: A community based cross-sectional study. BMC Pregnancy and Childbirth. 2017;**17**:70

[21] Okonofua F, Randawa A, Ogu R, Agholor K, Okike O, Abdus-salam RA, et al. Views of senior health personnel about quality of emergency obstetric care: A qualitative study in Nigeria. PLoS One. 2017;**12**(3):e0173414

Chapter 6

Forensic Midwifery

Sevde Aksu

Additional information is available at the end of the chapter

http://dx.doi.org/10.5772/intechopen.82222

Abstract

Midwifes who have an important role in "Mother and Child Health Services" in the world; is not included as a specialist area of forensic midwifery within the specialties of forensic sciences. We can see that studies of forensic midwifery are only implemented by forensic obstetric gynecology and forensic nursing. The midwife is one of the health personnel who can see the first forensic evidence, who first see the individual in most judicial cases, who first contacts the family or relatives, touches his or her equipment during the examination, and contacts the laboratory specimens taken individually. The purpose of this chapter is informing about content and characteristic of forensic midwifery that cannot find an application field in the world, attracting attention to forensic midwifery and stating that forensic midwifery can contribute to assessment of forensic apparitions.

Keywords: midwife, forensic midwifery, criminal cases, forensic midwifery roles, expertise

1. Introduction

When the health level of the countries and the effectiveness of the health services are evaluated; it is seen that the most important difference between the developing countries and the developed countries is in the field of "Mother and Child Health." The midwife is one of the most important members of the health care profession in terms of duties, powers and responsibilities [1].

By the World Health Organization (WHO); "A person trained to provide necessary care and counseling during pregnancy, childbirth and postpartum period, having normal births on his own responsibility, taking care of the newborn" [2]. According to the International Confederation of Midwives (ICM) the midwife; is a reliable and responsible professional who provides maternity care during pregnancy, childbirth and postnatal periods, performs birth on its own responsibility, provides neonatal care, and cooperates with women throughout life [3].

The aim of midwifery profession as a professional health discipline; advocate, practitioner, educator and researcher [4].

It should not be forgotten that midwives in the world have played a key role in the development of forensic nursing in recent years as a unifying and supporting role between medicine and the forensic. Forensic midwifery; the collection and protection of biological and physical evidence, the support and rehabilitation of victims and their relatives, the writing of a forensic report, the training and counseling of midwives/nursing services, and the role and responsibilities of preventing violence, as well as of victims of violence, trauma and other criminal events and trauma.

Despite the fact that the duties and responsibilities of forensic nurses in the world are defined within the scope of professional qualifications and ethical principles, there are no laws and regulations regarding forensic midwifery, so their fields of study cannot go beyond academic studies.

In this section we will examine the duties and responsibilities of the midwife who will meet forensic events.

2. Method

This chapter gives information about the scope and characteristics of forensic midwifery discipline, draws attention to forensic midwifery within the fields of forensic sciences and contributes significantly to the diagnosis, treatment and evaluation of forensic cases. This literature search included the midwives' duties and competences in terms of the factors affecting the health of women and pregnant women and having forensic dimensions (violence against women and pregnant women, etc.). Searches were conducted in PubMed, Cochrane and ScienceDirect, and included studies published in Turkey, English 2000–2018. Further studies were retrieved by detailed searches of the reference lists of identified articles.

3. Definition of forensic midwifery

Midwives, field work areas (obstetrics and gynecology clinics, child care and intensive care, child care centers, reproductive health clinics, family health centers, etc.) and legal responsibilities are taken into consideration.

The midwife is one of the health personnel who can see the first forensic evidence, who first see the individual in most judicial cases, who first contacts the family or relatives, touches his or her equipment during the examination, and contacts the laboratory specimens taken individually [5].

According to Hammer, during the forensic investigations where the midwives and nurses are not involved, the team members may not understand the emotional pain and trauma experienced by the victims when performing the legal procedures. Again according to Hammer, some characteristics of those who make medical examinations or who have the authority to impose legal sanctions are likely to be at risk of receiving improper care by the victims, their families and the factions. The approach of midwives to their emotional pain and trauma from the point of view of the mission of their profession is important in communicating with the victim and gathering evidence [6].

In this respect, the main duty of women and child health midwives in forensic events; it should not be forgotten that it will have important roles in history taking, physical examination, identification of evidence, collection of evidence, storage of evidence, provision of evidence protection chain, registration of evidence [7].

In this context forensic midwifery is; "Who monitors and reports traumatic injuries of victims (all age groups of women, pregnant women, postpartum, 0–6 age group) who are applying midwifery education and the knowledge and experience of clinical midwife practitioners using legal procedures for forensic medicine, the application area of forensic sciences working on the forensic cases, collecting evidence, analyzing the facts and evidence, taking part in the examination team of the sexual crime unit, working in a defendant and witness protection program, witnessing as an expert in the court and conducting scientific researches related to forensic midwifery studies" [8].

4. States showing characteristics of forensic midwifery

4.1. Violence against women

The midwife is in a far more strategic position, preventing the violence against women and the grounds for serving women in violent situations. Therefore, midwives have important duties in the early detection of cases of violence against women, and in the fact that women have acceptable ways of coping with the situation they are in, providing physical and psychological help [9].

WHO has listed the obligations of health workers in combating domestic violence against women as follows [10]:

- First, in the families where violence behaviors are experienced, the causes of violence and the assessment of possible risk factors.
- Emergency medical treatment for cases experiencing violent behavior and creation of social support environment.
- Police support in case of violence, participation of social workers, cooperation of health workers in cooperation with center help.

Midwife is a position that can provide adequate care for the victims, as well as nursing and emergency health nurses and public health nurses, in terms of domestic violence.

The first time the woman reports violence to her:

- The woman is examined, the trauma of the body is identified and the first intervention is made for the treatment.
- Make laboratory tests, radiological examinations and/or consultations as required.
- The hospital police are informed. The police station in the hospital starts the necessary judicial proceedings. This fact is considered a forensic case when the patient's health is impaired, when another person's careless, careless or negligent behavior or deliberate action is held responsible.
- The report records the examination findings.
- Fill in the registration form for domestic violence against women.
- If the patient decides on inpatient treatment, he will pay the appropriate service. If the hospital conditions are not sufficient for the patient and the physician considers it necessary, the patient will be referred to an advanced center. No patient can be discharged without urgent care without stabilization. In cases where necessary care is not provided, the patient and the relatives refer to the cause of the referral in detail and send the patient/injured with a suitable vehicle or ambulance after consultation with the interested physician in the hospital and the care guarantee.
- If the patient does not need to be hospitalized, the risk assessment is done. If the risk is not considered, the prescription is arranged and, if necessary, a follow-up plan is initiated by informing about the legal rights and the institutions that may be applied if there is a risk of violence again.
- If violence is considered to be a risk, the woman will be guided by the police to the institutions affiliated to the 'Social Services and Child Protection Agency' [11].

Midwives are also exposed to violence against women and violence against pregnancy in the work areas of nurses. Domestic violence during pregnancy; spouse/partner is defined as the threat of physical, sexual, economic or psychological/emotional violence applied by parents, siblings or other relatives to the pregnancy [12]. Increased maternal, fetal and newborn morbidity and mortality were associated with pregnancies exposed to physical, sexual and psychological violence during pregnancy. Domestic violence rates during pregnancy in international studies range from 1 to 20% due to cultural differences [13]. It shows that violence in marriage continues in pregnancy and that it is not obstructive to pregnancy in terms of physical violence [14]. According to WHO, it is inevitable for women to be exposed to violence during their pregnancies, as the search for domestic violence in communities cannot be done. Despite the prepared protocol, guidelines or special trainings on the subject, it is not routinely used by midwives, nurses and physicians [15].

In terms of midwives, the reasons for this situation; difficulties in defining violence, lack of information and education on family and pregnancy violence, lack of maintenance continuity, lack of time, recognition of social taboos and violence, evaluation of the evaluation outside of the tasks, authorities and responsibilities of the evaluation. However, the majority of women experiencing domestic violence in pregnancy acknowledge that the midwife profession is responsible for defining violence, providing first aid and adequate care. Midwives that working in women's health and maternity areas will create in their relationships with women; identification of the violence, evaluation of the incident, maintenance continuity and collection of evidence [13].

In this regard, midwives working in primary care should be able to identify risk groups and risk factors, particularly at the level of interrelationships between individuals, families and persons, to prevent domestic violence and direct women to supportive services to prevent the crisis [16].

Rape crimes show a ratio approaching 3% of all crimes per year in the World. The vast majority of those who have been attacked are concerned that the legal and medical systems may be inadequate and that this attack cannot be provoked by family members and society as evidenced by the family members and society, prefer to keep secret. In addition to the delays in the application of the forensic examination, the forensic examination equipment and devices may be inadequate, and the lack of knowledge and experience of the health care personnel may result in inadequate evidence [17]. A victim of sexual assault can cause tragic and traumatic events as well as almost sexual assault in a hospital where they are referred to on complaint. On the other hand, victims are kept in emergency services for hours, sometimes not available, and the fact that the clinics are referred to other cities or districts for reasons of inadequacy, while the judicial proceedings and the necessary evidence for the courts to be convened with appropriate methods must be meticulously and promptly collected. It is important to educate midwives who have been trained to ensure that the needs of all victims of child or women exposed to sexual assault in this stage are met accurately and completely.

The scope of the examination for sexual violence is also defined below:

- Informing the patient and taking his/her request.
- Taking the detailed history of the patient, including events that can be classified as sexual violence.
- Exact "top to bottom" physical examination.
- Detailed examination of the sexual organs and anus region.
- Recording and classification of identified injuries.
- Collection of identified medical samples for diagnostic purposes.
- Acquisition of forensic specimens.
- Influence of the obtained evidence in terms of the protection, packaging and delivery of necessary places.

- Investigation of psychological support possibilities and provision of magic (may be close to).
- Implementation of regulations regarding patient follow-up after examination.
- Bringing together all documents related to the patient and archiving.
- Preparation of medical and judicial reports (Authorized institutions) [18, 19].

According to Royal Midwifery College, the importance of ebelerin in the medical approach to violence victimized pregnancies is emphasized [20]. It also describes the approach of Ebecer from the forensic clinic staff as a professional healthcare provider to victims of sexual abuse according to the Guidelines for Forensic Clinical Approach to the Irish National Sexual Assault Victims [21].

"The role of health personnel in combating domestic violence against women and procedures to be implemented" is given for the personnel (doctors, nurses, nurses) who work in emergency services of institutions and hospitals in countries. However, these trainings should not be limited to the staff working in the emergency service but should be given to the women and children who work in the health field in all steps.

4.2. Substance dependency in pregnancy

Abuse of the substance is an important public health issue that concerns societies all over the world. There is also an increase in the use of drugs in females, such as smoking and alcohol. Cigarettes, alcohol and substance abuse are common in pregnant women who are particularly exposed to violence, and there are delays in taking prenatal care or applying to a health institution.

Substance use during pregnancy, maternal risks, fetal physical and mental problems increase, antenatal follow-up is also missing compared to other pregnancies. According to the 2005 National Survey on Drug Use and Health (NSDUH), among women between 15 and 44 years of reproductive age, the rate of substance use in pregnant women is 4% and in non-pregnant women is 10% [22]. It is estimated that between 20 and 30% of cigarette consumption, 15% of alcohol consumption, 3–10% of cannabis use, and 0.5–3% of cocaine use are among pregnant women [23]. When substance use in pregnancy is encountered, a multidisciplinary approach should be included in the patient evaluation of the midwives, together with the obstetrician, psychiatrist, public health specialist and pediatrician.

The most used items in pregnancy are alcohol, cocaine, opiates, amphetamines and cigarettes. Although the mechanism of fetal alcohol consumption, fetal pathophysiology and teratogenicity is not well known, alcohol itself or its metabolite acetaldehyde is considered to be one of the main factors affecting fetal development. The limit value that will lead to anomaly formation has not yet been determined. Alcohol affects the growth and development of the fetus by reducing protein synthesis [24].

Alcohol increases spontaneous abortion and stillbirth during pregnancy. Alcohol use in western societies is the leading cause of mental retardation. In the United States, 1 in 100 births is affected by it. If the mother consumes 4 drinks per day during pregnancy, the risk of fetal alcohol syndrome is 20%, 8% is 50% in domestic.

The definition of fetal alcohol syndrome (FAS) was first described in 1973. It contains a number of congenital anomalies that are associated with chronic alcohol use during pregnancy.

This syndrome should contain one or more items from each group of statements collected in the three main headings.

1. Intrauterine and/or postnatal growth retardation
2. Craniofacial anomalies
3. MSS dysfunctions [24, 25].

Alcohol dependence should be explained to the mother, frequent prenatal control should be done during the pregnancy, ultrasonographic examination should be repeated for follow-up. The patient should be included in counseling and rehabilitation programs.

Cocaine-induced cardiovascular effects in pregnancy are more pronounced due to increased progesterone. For the first time in 1985, the relationship between cocaine use and fetal anomaly in humans has begun to be investigated. One study shows an increase in the risk of minor anomalies by 1.6, major anomalies by 4.99, and urogenital anomalies by 6.5 times. Its use in pregnancy is a serious public health problem in terms of maternal, fetal and neonatal risks. The risk of placental abruption in cocaine-using pregnancies is significantly higher. This can be explained by reduced placental perfusion due to increased vasoconstriction in uterine vessels. Premature rupture of membranes, premature labor, intrauterine growth retardation, and the incidence of meconium and spontaneous abortion in amniotic fluid have also increased in cocaine-exposed pregnancies. Migraine attacks and hyperthermia are also detected during the mother's pregnancy. The fetus increases the risk of intrauterine cerebral infarction and urinary tract anomaly. Sleeping, eating disorders, hypertension, tremor can be seen in long-term follow-ups of these children. The rate of cognitive impairment in adolescents increased in these children. HIV and other infections may also be passed on to the child during maternal pregnancy [26].

Opiates, including morphine and codeine, are obtained from the poppy called *Papaver somniferum*. Opioid includes synthetic narcotics such as heroin, meperidine, fentanyl, propoxyphene and methadone. According to 2010 National Survey on Drug Use and Health, the rate of drug use in the United States is 4.4%, and heroin use is 0.1%. Perinatal complications of opioid use include intrauterine growth retardation, preterm delivery, fetal death, small head circumference, low Apgar score, meconium in amnios fluid, premature rupture of membranes and chorioamnionitis [27].

Amphetamines stimulate the sympathetic nervous system by increasing neurotransmitter release from the presynaptic terminal. Oral, iv or smoking can be taken. In a study involving women who did not use amphetamine in their pregnancy and those who did not, there was an increase in anemia, preterm birth, meconium amniotic fluid, and intrauterine growth retardation rates according to the control group. Its use in pregnancy poses significant risks to both mother and fetus. In addition, when children who were exposed to intrauterine amphetamine were examined, a 1-year delay was found in school achievement at 14–15 years of age [28].

About 250 million women smoke in the world. Nicotine and carbon monoxide adversely affect the development of fetus. Nicotine reduces vasoconstriction and uterine artery blood flow, while carbon monoxide reduces oxygen transport to fetal tissues. Circadian cyanide levels are higher in smokers and this substance has toxic effects on dividing cells. There is a relationship between low cigarette smoking, ectopic pregnancy, fetal growth retardation, ablative placenta, preterm birth, early rupture of membranes and low birth weight in pregnancy. Perinatal mortality is more than 150% [29].

Use of drugs by the health personnel and their awareness of the effects on the pregnant, fetus and newborn may enable them to be vigilant in this regard and take an active role in the policies to be set up for the prevention. In the determination of maternal substance and metabolites used in the baby, blood, urine, gaita saliva and hair analysis should be done besides mother's story. Although urine and blood tests provide information on the substance currently being used, hair analysis also gives an idea of the use of substances in the past. It is stated that newborn infants should not be satisfied with urine analysis but also meconium examination should be done. There are research findings indicating that substance metabolites have been detected in meconium of negative cases [29].

Knowledge of the characteristics of women with substance abuse is important for early detection and intervention of risk groups. These features:

- Women who have not had a positive relationship with their parents.
- Those who have not seen a positive parental role model.
- Those who have lived in an environment where domestic violence has been practiced.
- Those who have experienced physical, emotional and sexual abuse and neglect in the family environment.
- Parents are drug addicts.
- In marriage, they are abused by their wives. Detection of pregnant women in early period and pregnant women using substance should be taken into intensive prenatal care program and substance use in pregnancy should be informed about adverse effects on fetus and mother.

5. Forensic midwifery roles and responsibilities

Forensic midwifery is a new concept and is a concept used together with medicine, law and criminology. It can also be seen as an example of innovation in terms of expanding the roles of midwives in the field of women's health and safety.

In this respect, the tasks of forensic midwifery; suspicion of violence against women and children, identification of statements, gathering of evidence, crisis intervention, and directing the necessary actions.

In this regard, midwives can work in emergency rooms, suicide prevention centers, rape crisis centers, crime scene investigations, death investigations, prisons, law offices and forensic pathology laboratories and at the same time as expert witnesses in court [17].

While the forensic midwife performs its roles and responsibilities, she is accompanied by a forensic team consisting of forensic scientists, forensic scientists, psychologists, gynecologists, social workers, members of the judiciary (judges, prosecutors, lawyers) and security members (police, gendarmerie) can work. In addition, forensic nurses can work with Forensic Medicine Institution, Forensic Medicine Institutes and expert institutions [30–33].

5.1. Collection of physical evidence

Evidence collection is one of the processes that are important in a review and the midwife is part of this process. The midwives should be sure that nothing has been missed by taking part in each of the techniques and stages of evidence collection. Criminal cases such as murder, rape, rape, traffic accidents are first applied to emergency services. Forensic midwives are inadvertently served by the investigator/investigator when a victim is brought to the emergency service. At this stage, the midwives evaluate and record all the data about the victim and the medical conditions, bruising, cuts, lacerations and places that require treatment. Forensic examinations may be assisted by civil servants in the case of saliva, sirens, lead, the removal of bullets from the body, and the evaluation of clothes and items of the victim for further examination. When physical evidence is collected, gloves must be worn to minimize contamination and to observe basic techniques and procedures. Anything remaining at the scene must be collected, and evidence that DNA analysis can be performed should be obtained by appropriate techniques.

They have more favorable conditions than other healthcare team members, such as having nursing nurses on the collection, preservation and storage of medical evidence. The midwives' sensitive attitudes about the collection, preservation and protection of forensic evidence provide for the identification and reporting of healthier and richer evidence in the judicial investigation process [34–36].

5.2. Record of evidence

It must be ensured that the medical records that are held are legally available. It should be avoided that the terminology is such as to ignore the evidence. The victim must use his/her expressions directly when taking the statement. The prescribed medical treatments should be recorded, the bruises and injuries should be indicated by color, number and size [34–36].

5.3. Storage of evidence

Health care institutions should develop procedures for recording and tracking suspect deaths. Standard practice procedures should be developed and the team should know how to act in a suspicious situation. All health professionals should know how to protect evidence and how to behave in judicial cases and follow these procedures [34–36].

5.4. Provision of evidence protection chain

As you walk through the evidence, each person should record the date and time they opened the package. In this way, the disappearance of evidence can be prevented. You should be asked to write the name, surname, job and department you are evaluating. The duration of the evidence chain and evidence must be kept as short as possible. Precautions must be taken to ensure that the evidences are not altered and that they are not affected by external conditions when the collected evidence is sent into or out of the institution [34–36].

5.5. Testimony in court

Forensic examinations can be witnessed in courts. If the midwife is called as a witness to a court; should be consistent with the written statements and the resulting physical evidence collected. The use of improper terminology can make it more difficult to enlighten. The terms used in the emblem should be in a way that everyone understands, and the possible causes and mechanisms of injury should be understood and explained appropriately. It should be avoided to give an idea about the issues outside the field of expertise. By following these steps and collecting the appropriate evidence, the victim's fear of the legal system can be avoided [37, 38].

In this context, we can list the specific areas where judges can fulfill their roles and responsibilities as follows;

5.6. Clinical forensic midwifery

Midwives working in emergency services intervene especially in victims of trafficking or victims. Forensic midwives working in this location are responsible for the care and treatment of the patient during the period between the hospital and the discharge of the patient, the collection and storage of the forensic evidence, the accurate and complete medical records, the taking of the prosecutor's office and court order for biological and chemical examinations, to be properly removed and stored, and to collect information and evidence in accordance with the relevant regulations [30, 32, 34, 37, 38].

5.7. Sexual assault examination midwifery

They are specializing in special care and treatment for victims of sexual assault. Among his tasks are; to investigate sexually transmitted diseases and to advise the victim on this issue, to collect, store and transmit the forensic evidence, to help the victim, to evaluate the injuries, to take medical narratives, to make physical examinations, to record criminal information.

The legal process midwife should be a professional who is helping the family in this abusive process, treating medical records and photos in child abuse, monitoring criminals in hospitals, watching victims in courts or nursing homes [31, 32, 34].

5.8. Pediatric forensic midwifery

This field of midwife is responsible for monitoring the possibility of events such as acceptance and evaluation of child abuse and neglect cases, treatment, referral to preventive service units, domestic violence, battered child syndrome and sudden child death, monitoring and rehabilitation of the victim. Midwives are responsible for providing care to children who need help with issues such as abuse, neglect and violations of human rights. While they should provide care for children, it should be carefully assessed to see if there are any signs and symptoms of children experiencing ill-treatment [36, 37].

5.9. Obstetrics and gynecology forensic midwifery

This field-based midwife is responsible for taking and recording accurate and complete stories about the physical and psychological trauma of women, domestic violence, assessment of substance abuse in pregnancies, general follow-up of pregnant women allegedly traumatized, low, early or stillbirth- and as a witness when necessary [36, 37].

5.10. Midwifery in rape crisis centers

The nurse working in this area is required to make a visit to sexually assaulted persons, to ensure that evidence is collected and maintained in a proper and appropriate manner, to provide information to the victim and his relatives at every stage of the treatment, to ensure that the victim is safe to leave the center, to serve him in the rehabilitation and presentation of the place to stay at the center until he comes from the center [36, 37].

5.11. Expertise

Forensic midwives should be able to function in the application of neglect and malpractice and medical records.

6. Discussion

Midwives' activities are medical interventions and the conditions of activity and legal compliance are the same. Midwives who provide health care are the persons who are trained to provide medical services, are authorized to take medical care in the area where they are qualified and responsible for this action. Therefore, the important duties of the midwife in the diagnosis, treatment, rehabilitation of the factors that affect the health of women and pregnant (such as violence, rape, dependence) and the transfer of information between institutions (such as forensic institutions) are determined by the laws and regulations of the countries. The concept of forensic midwifery is important in terms of the effective use of the roles of advocates, practitioners, educators and researchers. Therefore, although the duties and responsibilities of the forensic nurses in the world are defined within the scope of occupational characteristics and ethical principles, they should add studies on the forensic midwives to the theoretical and practical applications of midwives working in the field of women's health.

7. Conclusion

The addition of forensic midwifery to the undergraduate and postgraduate midwife education curriculum, the issuance of necessary laws and regulations on the subject and the regulation of scientific research, courses and seminars will contribute to the development of forensic midwifery.

In this respect, forensic midwives, midwives with licensed professional licenses should be formed. In addition, after attending regular undergraduate midwifery trainings, they must become specialized and participate in courses in the field of forensic sciences and must be trained on issues such as the protection of physical evidence, identification of injury, and detection of laws.

As a new area of expertise, forensic midwifery serves as a bridge to closing the gap between law and medicine. The need for a forensic midwife will become more and more likely to perceive and accept the critical and important role of the forensic midwife in establishing the link between civil servants, lawyers, other health professionals, the law and the health system within the justice system [38].

Author details

Sevde Aksu

Address all correspondence to: sevde.c@gmail.com

Midwifery Department, Health Science Faculty, Balikesir University, Turkey

References

[1] Taşkın L. Birth and Women's Health Nursing. 2nd ed. Ankara: Sistem Ofset Typography; 2012. pp. 8-9

[2] Arslan H, Krahan N, Çam Ç. Midwifery effects on nature and form of birth. Maltepe Üniversitesi Hemşirelik Bilim ve Sanatı Dergisi. 2008;**1**(2):54

[3] International Confederation of Midwives. The Hague, The Netherlands: The philosophy and model of midwifery care Laan van Meerdervoor [Internet]. 2003. Available from: http://www.internationalmidwives.org/assets/uploads/documents/CoreDocuments/CD2005_001%20ENG%20Philosophy%20and%20Model%20of%20Midwifery %20Care.pdf [Accessed: Jun 18, 2018]

[4] Jones SR, Symon A. Ethics in Midwifery. 2nd ed. Edinburgh: Elsevier Limited, Mosby. 2000. pp. 3-187

[5] Savaş H. Responsibilities Arising from Medical Intervention of Health Workers and Health Care Institutions. 2nd ed. Ankara: Seçkin Bookstore; 2007. 47 p

[6] Hammer R. Caring İn forensic nursing: Expanding the holistic model Journal of Psychosocial Nursing and Mental Health Services. 2000;**38**(11):18-24. https://doi.org/10.3928/0279-3695-20001101-09

[7] Hancı H. Forensic nursing. Türkiye Klinikleri Hemşirelik Bilimleri Dergisi. 2003;**1**:51

[8] Aksu S. Forensic midwifery. Henoch-Schönlein Purpura. 2017;**4**(3):277-284. DOI: 10.17681/hsp.306089

[9] Arabacı L, Karadağlı A. Developing scale to recognize the signs of violence against women by midwives and nurses. Sağlık ve Toplum. 2006;**16**(2):101-112

[10] World Health Organisation (WHO). Guidelines for Medico-Legal Care for Victims of Sexual Violence [Internet]. Geneva: WHO; 2003. Available from: www.who.int/violence_injury_prevention/publications/violence/med_leg_guidelines/en/ [Accessed: Jun 18, 2018]

[11] Çifçi Ö. Assessment of hopelessness, depression and reproductive health status of women who applied to shelters due to violence they experienced [thesis]. İstanbul: Marmara Üniversitesi Sağlık Bilimleri Enstitüsü; 2009

[12] Finnbogadóttir H, Dykes A. Midwives' awareness and experiences regarding domestic violence among pregnant women in southern Sweden. Midwifery. 2012;**28**(2):181-189

[13] Antonella N, Giuseppina P, Zobbi V. Midwifery, domestic violence during pregnancy: midwives' experiences. Midwifery. 2015;**31**:498-504

[14] Tezcan S, Yavuz S, Tunçkanat H. Domestic violence against women and health results. In: T.C. Prime Ministry General Directorate of Women's Status (KGSM): Research on Domestic Violence against Women in Turkey. Ankara: Elma Teknik Basım Matbabacılık; 2009. pp. 71-82

[15] Lawoko S, Sanz S, Helström L, Castren M. Screening for intimate partner violence against women in healthcare Sweden: Prevalence and determinants. ISRN Nursing. 2012:7 p (Article ID 510692). DOI: 10.5402/2011/510692

[16] Akın A. Duties and responsibilities of healthcare staff in the fight against domestic violence against women [Internet]. 2008. Available from: https://kadininstatusu.aile.gov.tr/data/542a8e0b369dc31550b3ac30/02%20kyais%20mucadelede%20saglik%20hizmetleri.pdf [Accessed: Jun 18, 2018]

[17] Gökdoğan M, Erkol Z. Forensic nursing in Bolu, Turkey: A survey. Journal of Clinical Forensic Medicine. 2005;**12**:14-17

[18] Yayla D. Knowledge, attitudes and behavior levels of physicians and nurses related to violence against women [thesis]. İstanbul: Marmara Üniversitesi Sağlık Bilimleri Enstitüsü; 2009

[19] National action plan to combat domestic violence against women 2007-2010. A project to combat domestic violence against women [Internet]. 2009. Available from: http://kadininstatusu.aile.gov.tr/data/54296cb3369dc32358ee2c51/Kad%C4%B1na%20

Y%C3%B6nelik%20Aile%20%C4%B0%C3%A7i%20%C5%9Eiddet%20Ulusal%20 Eylem%20Plan%C4%B1%20(2012_2015).pdf [Accessed: Jun 18, 2018]

[20] Gill M, Loraine B, Alison H, Susan B. Midwives' perceptions and experiences of routine enquiryfor domestic violence. British Journal of Obstetrics and Gynaecology. 2003; **110**:744-752

[21] National SATU Guidelines Development Group Recent rape sexual assault national guidelines on referral and forensic clinical examination in Ireland. Support Nurse/ Midwife Role [Internet]. 2010. Available from: http://www.garda.ie/Documents/User/ recent%20rape%20%20sexual%20assault%20-%20national%20guidelines%20on%20 referral%20and%20forensic%20clinical%20examination%202010.pdf [Accessed: Jun 18, 2018]

[22] Bhuvaneswar CG, Chang G, Epstein LA, Stern TA. Cocaine and opioid use during pregnancy: Prevalence and management. Prim care companion. The Journal of Clinical Psychiatry. 2008;**10**:59-65. DOI: 10.4088/PCC.v10n0110

[23] Lamy S, Thibaut F. Psychoactive substance use during pregnancy: A review. Encephale. 2010;**36**(1):33-38

[24] Atasü T, Benian A. The Effects of Addictive Substances on the Fetus. İstanbul: Nobel Tıp Kitabevi; 2000. pp. 461-465

[25] Lui S, Terplan M, Smith EJ. Psychosocial interventions for women enrolled in alcohol treatment during pregnancy. Cochrane Database of Systematic Reviews. 2008;**16**:CD006753

[26] Cain MA, Bornick P, Whiteman V. The maternal, fetal, and neonatal effects of cocaine exposure in pregnancy. Clinical Obstetrics and Gynecology. 2013;**56**:124-132

[27] National Institute on Drug Abuse. Commonly abused prescription drugs [Internet]. 2011. Available from: https://www.drugabuse.gov/sites/default/files/rx-drugs-placemat-508c-10052011.pdf [Accessed: Jun 18, 2018]

[28] Phupong V, Darojn D. Amphetamine abuse in pregnancy: The impact on obstetric outcome. Archives of Gynecology and Obstetrics. 2007;**276**:167-170. DOI: 10.1007/ s00404-007-0320-x

[29] Cimete G. Effect of substance use on pregnancy, mother, fetus and newborn. Atatürk Üniversitesi Hemşirelik Yüksekokulu Dergisi. 2002;**5**(1):68-71

[30] Lynch VA. Forensic nursing science: Global strategies in health and justice. Egyptian Journal of Forensic Sciences. 2011;**1**:69-76

[31] Pınar R, Bahar MT. Emergency services and forensic nursing. Turkiye Klinikleri Hemşirelik Bilimleri Dergisi. 2011;**3**:45-54

[32] Özden D, Yıldırım N. Approach of forensic nurses. Hacettepe Üniversitesi Sağlık Bilimleri Fakültesi Hemşirelik Dergisi. 2009;**16**:73-81

[33] Rape Crisis Centers [Internet]. 2009. Available from: http://www.stgm.org.tr/tr/icerik/detay/tecavuz-kriz-merkezleri. [Accessed: Jun 18, 2018]

[34] Eşiyok B, Yelken N, Hancı H. Forensic nursing and the situation in Turkey. Adli Psikiyatri Dergisi. 2004;**1**(3):5-10

[35] Abdool NNT, Brysiewicz P. A descrıptıon of the forensıc nursıng role in emergency departments in urban. South Afrıca Journal of Emergency Nursıng. 2009;**35**:1

[36] Yost B, Stevens, S. Crackıng the case: Your role in forensic nursing [Internet]. 2010. Available from: http://npic.orst.edu/RMPP/rmpp_main2a.pdf [Accessed: Jun 18, 2018]

[37] Sunmaz D, Başbakkal Z, Bolışık B. Working areas of the forensic nurse. Adli Bilimler Dergisi (Turkish Journal of Forensic Sciences). 2009;**7**(3):42-47

[38] Charman L, Miller C, Leadingham R, McKean M. Forensic nursing: An emerging competency for contemporary practice. Teaching and Learning in Nursing. 2009;**5**(3):98-103